Overcoming Rejection

How to Create a Plan That Both Empowers

(Steps the Believer Must to Take to Win the Battle of Approval)

Willie Condon

Published By **Bella Frost**

Willie Condon

Overcoming Rejection: How to Create a Plan That Both Empowers (Steps the Believer Must to Take to Win the Battle of Approval)

ISBN 978-1-77485-738-0

No part of this guidebook shall be reproduced in any form without permission in writing from the publisher except in the case of brief quotations embodied in critical articles or reviews.

Legal & Disclaimer

Table of contents

Introduction

Everyone is aware that rejection can be a sour note. The feeling of rejection makes you question your self-esteem and abilities. You feel as if you're not enough. The agony of rejection can definitely crush your confidence and sever you to your center.

Humans are naturally social. We all want to be valued and accepted. Rejection is a slap in the face to our desire to be loved and acknowledged. Being told that we're not enough is a sign that we're not accepted as a member of the group, and this causes deep fear and hurt in our hearts. The terrible pain that rejection can inflict on us can trigger a deep-seated fear of rejection for many people.

Unfortunately, a lot of people are controlled by fear of rejection. They create safe, small box of limitations around themselves, and do not consider the risk required to establish a company or even approach a gorgeous woman. Their lives are limited and they miss out on wonderful opportunities because of their fears. The fear of rejection is an effective way of keeping people from taking crucial chances and avoiding life. This is an embarrassment. You're not gaining acceptance by settling in a secure area and trying to avoid the rejection. The fact that rejection is a painful experience does not mean that you must be a slave to stay out of it.

As with all fears, the worry about being rejected is one that you have to be able to overcome. Being open to rejection is one method to conquer the anxiety of it. Learning to view rejection as an opportunity to learn instead of a painful event, can make you able to accept rejection with confidence because you realize that it's nothing to be scared of.

It is impossible to be completely resistant to rejection. It happens and is a element of the human condition. It is impossible to avoid rejection. Instead, it's best to accept the fact that rejection will occur in your lifetime, possibly numerous times. It's not something that can be avoided or prevented completely regardless of how you do.

You can however increase the chances of getting yes. How you portray you to people, and how you conduct conversations or engage with people you love can impact your life's success. You're less likely to be rejected if your use specific methods to approach others that show confidence, for example, and presenting yourself with confidence. If you can make people feel that the offer you make to them is just too great to refuse and you are able to get acceptance.

It is also possible to alter the way you feel about rejection. If you can remove the fear and terror that comes with rejection out of your thoughts The fear of rejection will not as scary anymore. You can utilize rejection to your advantage. Rejection is a opportunity to grow as a person, and increase the value you provide romantic partners or business potential partners. If you change the way you view rejection and the way you think about it, you will be able to eliminate the anxiety associated with it. With no fear of rejection, you'll no longer be scared to try your hand at it and to achieve new goals.

Fear can be destroyed when you cease to take rejection as personal. It is also destroyed when you cease giving it the power to rule you. It is okay to accept that rejection can be painful however, you do not need to let your fear of suffering dictate the way you live your life. Instead, accept the fact that rejection is a normal part of life , refusing to let it have any influence or power over your choices.

It's what it is to be rejected-proof. If you are wearing a bullet-proof vest, there is just as high a chance of be targeted as someone who doesn't have having a vest on. However, the bullets bounce off your body and don't penetrate the skin. This is in line that you are able to be rejection-proof. There is always the possibility of rejection. However, rejection will pass through you and you'll be capable of moving on without the emotional damage that rejection causes certain people. Rejection won't kill your self-esteem.

This book is the best guide for becoming reject-proof. You will be taught how to look at rejection in a different way so that you can deal with rejection in a positive way. Also, you'll learn how ways to decrease your chances of being rejected as well as increase the likelihood of getting accepted. The fear of rejection will no longer be able to reach you after you have applied the principles throughout this text. This means that you will be able to take on aspects of your life you had never thought of doing before. You'll be more inclined to take on big chances because you're not scared of the results. When you take on this risk, you might be able to transform you life around to be more than you could have ever thought possible.

Chapter 1: The Reasons Why Rejection Hurts

It's not a secret that rejection is painful. What is the reason why rejection causes people to feel so badly? The pain of rejection is so intense that people tend to shy away from it, just as they would shun the heat of a stove or torture device. People are hesitant to face the pain in their own way, suggesting that they are programmed to avoid rejection.

When you feel rejected when you are rejected, the pain centers in your brain are activated. Similar neurons which are activated when you fall on your leg are activated when you're being not accepted. In essence, your brain feels the same physical pain when confronted with rejection. Scientists who placed subjects under MRI devices and asked them to recall an experience of rejection, observed the same neural activation in brains that is seen within the minds of patients experiencing physical pain.

The hurt of rejection is extremely real and incredibly painful. It is felt throughout your body. A small, intimate friendship that falls apart or an entire group of strangers who snub you at a bar can trigger a deep feeling of disapproval.

In addition to feeling dejected and resentful, you may also be shamed of how damaged you feel. It is difficult not to accept that something that tiny could make you feel so hurt. There is a chance that you don't know why even the tiniest rejections are so painful. You may feel more vulnerable when you receive tiny rejections because you don't know how major rejection could be.

If you suffer a severe rejection, you'll feel like you're incapable of functioning. It may be as if you've lost someone very dear to you, and believe that you've lost a portion of your self. Being rejected by your family, or the society at large can cause you to feel a gnarly discomfort. The blow to your self-esteem is similar to the damage on your body.

The human brain deals with refusal with exactly the same intensity as physical trauma since the brain of humans is wired to depend on the approval of others. Being accepted by fellow human beings is as crucial to the brain as protecting one's physical and health. This brain reaction to rejection is an consequence of the hunter-gatherer era of human history, where humans were required to band together in order to survive. Being part of the herd meant your odds of survival were greater since you had other people helping to detect and defend yourself from threats. Not being part of the herd meant you were on your own to defend yourself and would not be able to last for long in to spot and fight off danger on your own. In the dark caveman times there were all kinds of dangers that were present in the form of wild animals to natural disasters. Being able to take care of yourself during the caveman era was almost impossible without the help of a team.

The human brain therefore became sensitive to rejection and experience the same fear as physical assaults against the human body. If the brain detects that it is being rejected it is programmed to respond immediately by causing intense discomfort. The purpose of this discomfort is to force humans to change their behavior that they are accepted a part of the herd, and to improve the chances of survival. This is the reason people tend to adhere to the norms of society and social norms, in order to avoid being excluded by the herd.

Human brains are in a state of being wired to want for a partner to pass on genetic information. Find a partner who would like to be your partner is crucial for your brain. If you suffer from rejection for love it is natural to be damaged because the chances of passing down your genes are slowed. This is also stressful and painful for the brain, which is the reason it is so difficult and embarrassing.

It is extremely challenging without the help of other people. However, it's not as difficult to live by yourself as it used to be. The fear of being on your own is very present for humans, however. The brain's hardwiring is not changing. Our brain has changed extremely slowly, while society has morphed very rapidly. The brain isn't given enough time to adjust to the latest social trends. So the brain will retain old ways of thinking that are no longer serving people effectively.

In the end, we generally have to endure the deep and natural fear of being rejected as a relic of the past times. Rejection fear is a fundamental aspect of every human. It's difficult for many to bear the hurt of rejection, and they are naturally inclined to stay away from it. But it isn't always feasible. The pain of rejection isn't gone but it's often a traumatic aspect of life. In the world of romance and business Rejection is a frequent occurrence. It's inevitable unless you plan to sit in your home all daylong, not doing anything.

The truth is that a lot of the hurt caused by rejection is caused by self-inflicted. Though rejection can be painful however, it becomes overwhelming when one ponders the incident and decides to let it harm their self-esteem, and causes them to doubt themselves. The feeling of being rejected is powerful enough to make a person question their feeling of belonging, which can lead to self-doubt that is utterly resentful. Being rejected as a member of the crowd can cause someone to question their value as an individual. Being disregarded can cause a lot of emotional bruising. Many people are prone to acting self-destructive and aggravate their feelings by considering rejection as a matter of seriousness believing that one rejection is a sign of everything wrong with their own.

People who are rejected tend to think about their own anxieties. If someone has a lot of anxiety, degree of fear The first thing they will think of when they're rejected is that they're insufficient and unloved by the world. When they try to figure out what went wrong that led to their rejection in order to adapt their behavior to fit to the norm, they often consider their own fears as the reason for the rejection. "I have been rejected because I'm overweight." "I are too pushy to get anyone to like me." "I don't an excellent painter which is why people don't want to display my work in their gallery." Although those aren't the main reasons for rejection, many people blame themselves for their failures. It makes the pain of rejection to the point that those who are rejected let it rub on their most sensitive spots.

The insecurities of people are usually triggered from an early age. They may have been engrained into the brain of a child by an abusive parent or a peer or learned through media. Whatever the reason for insecurity, no matter how it began they can make people insane. Many people notice their weaknesses way more than other people. A rejection can make imperfections appear even more glaring. Rejection based on a weakness, for instance, an intimate rejection due to weight, can provide positive reinforcement for insecurity which suggests that it's an actual flaw, and hinders the person from being accepted and loved by other people. This is why rejection can exacerbate insecurity.

The feeling of rejection is as physical pain. However, it can also trigger flashes of anger and mood changes. A lot of rejection can cause permanent mood changes including depression. Concentrating on your anxieties about rejection could make the mental turmoil worse. it.

Psychopaths such as Ted Bundy are examples of people who let rejection make them crazy. They are driven by the anger spurts and the hurt that rejection can result in. Instead of healing in a quiet place until healing People who are hurt tend to react violently and violently. The extreme reactivity to rejection is a prime illustration of how severely and deeply rejection can harm people. While the majority of people do not take action on the feelings that result from rejection, it does trigger extremely powerful emotions and violent thoughts.

A time-long experience of rejection may result in two different impacts on someone. It could either make someone more resistant against rejection, making them a rejection-proof person, or it could make someone frightened and reluctant to live a full life. The way you react to rejection is entirely dependent on you. You decide how you'd prefer you to allow your mind process rejection. It is definitely more beneficial to let your rejection mold you into a better person. Transforming the negative feeling of rejection into a positive experience will make you feel more positive and make you an expert at dealing with any rejection that comes your way in the near future.

You are able to decide how to approach rejection. Even with the force of your instincts there is a way to train your brain to not follow your instincts in the face of rejection. You can prepare yourself for the fear of rejection and also teach yourself to view the rejection as an opportunity to learn by requiring yourself to maintain an optimistic view of it. You can also train your brain to stop causing hurt on yourself.

With time, by maintaining an optimistic attitude and not ignoring the fear of rejection you can teach your brain to think about rejection in a different way than it would normally. Your brain is naturally attracted to avoid rejection due to the fear of rejection however, you can overcome the strength of your emotions and teach your brain to accept rejection in a way that isn't life-threatening. In the beginning, you'll have to force yourself to cheer at first, but eventually it will become routine which will allow your brain to naturally accept rejection with no fear. Once you reach this level of comprehension it is then possible to live your life fully and unhindered by the hurt of rejection.

Learn from the writer Jia Jiang. Jiang set out on a quest of being rejected 100 days. Instead of letting the 100 rejections dampen his enthusiasm of life Jiang rather decided that he would never never be rejected. He embraced his fears of rejection and committed himself to overcoming it successfully. He utilized rejection as a way to examine the person he is and also to learn to accept rejection in order to be more successful later on.

There is no need to be adamant about seeking rejection for the duration of a hundred days however, you might be able to make use of rejection as a way of getting ready you can avoid being rejected in the near future. Let rejection help you grow and help you grow instead of weakening you and make you fall down.

It all boils down to the way you view rejection. This will be the subject for the next section.

Chapter 2: Rethink Your Perspective On Rejection

The first step in conquering your fear of rejection is to change the way you think about rejection. Change your attitude towards rejection could make it less intimidating and frightening for you. You can make your brain not stop at the fear of being rejected, even though it is innate and throughout all humans. In the end, you'll be able overcome your fears and take on the chances that bring life to. You'll be amazed at the things you can achieve through life when you do not allow fear to keep you from doing something.

If you change your perspective on rejection, you will be able to change your attitude towards rejection from one that is based on fear to one of acceptance. Positive acceptance is when acceptance of rejection is fact of life and recognize that you can't resist it. Also, it means that you start to take rejection in a positive perspective, and focus on overcoming rejection and the difficulties it creates, instead of trying to avoid it.

Through this improved relationship with rejection, it ceases to be a barrier to your daily life. It becomes an element of your life that you're capable of overcoming. The fear of being rejected can be replaced with problem solving and creativity. This will lead you to success.

Accept Rejection

There will be times when you are rejected in the course of your life. It is inevitable to be subject to it. Therefore, you must learn to cope with it. Accepting the fact that you will be rejected is essential to overcome the fear of rejection.

Unfortunately, you aren't going to be everybody's cup of tea. There will be those who do not like your style. There will be those who don't believe in the things you offer and who are likely to decline your offer in romance or business. The rejection rate is higher in certain industries like when you're launching your own business and looking for investors, or trying to sell music, a book or some other creative venture. You do your best to give something you're proud of however, others don't see any worth in it.

It's not pleasant however, it's to be accepted. It's also acceptable to meet people you think are attractive. This does not mean you're a horrible person or an unlikable person that nobody likes. It is more likely that you're facing a lot of competition around the globe. You need to realize that rejection is a human response to being overwhelmed. With so many offers pouring into the market from all directions People are expected to be selective in the places they invest their time and effort. They can't devote all of their time and energy to everyone. So, they are likely to turn down a lot of the offers they are offered. If you're rejected, it does not mean you're worthless. It was just that you were approached by an individual who did not recognize the value in you, due to reasons not your fault.

It is very likely that you will be rejected at some point throughout your life. But there's also the possibility that you'll be accepted. If you are beginning to worry about rejection, you should think "There is a fifty-fifty probability that I'll be either rejected or accepted. If I don't try and never discover what the outcome will be. It's a good idea to attempt."

If you approach risk in this way it helps you avoid being afraid of rejection, which causes in the majority of people. Accepting that rejection is inevitable can help you prepare yourself for it. You can develop a Plan B. It's not an end in itself for you when you take the time to consider alternative solutions. It's always a good idea to plan out what you'd do if you are disqualified. Recognizing rejection can help you start thinking about solutions for the rejection.

If you are prepared to accept the fact that rejection is inevitable it is unlikely to be so shocked by it. The aspect of surprise will most likely to shatter your confidence. You think it will be the case but if it doesn't it is a long descent from your high of self-confidence. However, if you go into something with the expectation of a rejection You won't be so shocked by the outcome since you won't be embarrassed when your belief of acceptance turns out to be untrue.

Take into consideration all possible outcomes

It's possible to never make a decision since you can only imagine one result: a firm no. However, no regardless of how well you are familiar with someone, you will never be able to discern minds. There are many more possibilities that are more than a simple no.

Think about the various possibilities. You might hear the word "yes. You might hear a possible. It could be heard an "no.

Then, think about the best way to respond to every possible reaction. If you are hearing a possibility then you should begin to sell yourself to transform that possible into the affirmative. In contrast you might consider a different strategy in the event that you hear a no. What happens if you get that yes? Then you must start making plans for your future!

Thinking about the various possible results of your idea can provide a sensation of suspense. This creates a sense of suspense. will be looking at the possibilities of what happens when you decide to take a risk.

This will encourage you to attempt something new without anxiety.

View Rejection as a Progression

A great blog on rejection, which is titled "Dumb Little Man," gives the advice: See rejection as a progression. This is a great suggestion. It is possible to develop a mindset which transforms negative thoughts into something positive experience. Naturally, rejection is painful and can be a drain on your soul. However, instead of getting buried in sorrow it is possible to feel better faster through a positive shift in your thoughts.

A lot of people consider rejection to be the result of a regression. It's easy to think that you are working for an answer and when you get a non, efforts have been in vain and you need to go back to where you started. This could be an experience that feels like the process of regress.

But , it's not about simply a couple of steps back. Rejection is a sign that you took one step towards the future. In reality, rejection is a way to move towards your goals in life.

Thinking about rejection in this way can help to alleviate some of the suffering caused by rejection.

The rejection of someone is a positive step in your life due to the fact that you made it to present someone an idea, or suggestion. You've made enough progress to conquer the fear of being rejected. Even if your plan was rejected doesn't negate any factual evidence that suggests you attempted.

It is also a sign of progress because it will teach you lessons and allow you to grow as an individual. Each time you encounter an unwelcome rejection, you learn some things about what does not work. You discover ways you can improve the quality of what you offer. You will be able to identify blind spots and mistakes in your plans by collaborating with others.

Sometimes an idea or plan is perfect until you explain it to someone else who exposes flaws you did not notice. If someone critiques you for your personality and you begin to realize aspects of your own personality that you require to alter. Although recognizing the shortcomings in your work can be a stinging experience but it can also help you to look at the areas you could make better.

It is not a good idea to be influenced by or alter yourself based on the opinions of other people. You can however use the views of other people to gain knowledge about how you can enhance your own work and projects. Sometimes, you may not have the same view of yourself and your work as other people have. Others may offer insightful insight into the things you could change.

The reality is that hearing that you're not perfect can be very painful. However, you can lessen your pain by taking the negative feedback of other people to make improvements to yourself instead of beating yourself up.

Don't take it personally

It is important not to consider every rejection as a personal attack. Sometimes, rejection is due to reasons that have nothing to do with have anything to do with your actions. The person who is responsible for the rejection is not accountable for every rejection you encounter.

There are times when people face other situations in their lives that stop them from accepting a proposal. A gorgeous woman you meet may be married, or she may be too timid to speak to you. Business prospects who turn away from your collaboration proposal could be having financial difficulties in a closed-door environment and can't afford to join you. The publisher who writes you a rejection notice may not be able additional books in that financial quarter or the publishing firm is specialized in the same genre as the book you created.

Don't ever think that rejection is solely based on your shortcomings as human beings. The fact that someone does not like you or your work , it does not mean that you are lacking anything valuable to offer the world. The fact that they reject you is likely to speak about them, not you. There are many reasons someone might be unable to accept you but don't be a victim and think that the rejection is solely due to you.

You could save yourself lots of heartache when you stop thinking of rejection as an attack on your personal life.

Rejection Doesn't Always Have to Be Because of your faults

In the first chapter I discussed the fact that rejection is often painful because people blame themselves for it. The majority of the pain caused by rejection is caused by self-inflicted. The self-inflicted hurt is a result of the human tendency to translate rejection into a assertion about the flaws in our internal lives. People are inclined to seek reasons why they were rejected, which leads them to imagine the reasons of their rejection. Most often, people see their fears as real and believe that the reason for rejection is an issue they perceive within themselves.

It's not a good idea to believe this. You're not an expert on mind reading, so do not try to understand the thoughts of those who do not like you. You will never know the reason for rejection until someone says it outright. Thus, you can't be sure that the deepest anxieties are to blame.

Most of the time, you only discern the things you're not confident about. You magnify small flaws, perhaps thinking of flaws that aren't at all. In the end, you believe that you are a victim of obvious, serious flaws which is something that no one else has. Your self-magnified flaws are likely not the reason for the rejection you feel.

If you realize that rejection always happens due to self-absorbed imperfections, you can reduce the amount rejection is a pain.

Rejection Today Doesn't Mean Rejection In the future

A single rejection, or multiple rejections, doesn't mean you'll be rejected for ever. The number of rejections that you experience will not affect the probability of fifty percent to be accepted by each future endeavor. If you keep trying and succeed, you might be successful.

Many authors go through numerous rejections before finding their first big break. Even actors with the biggest names have struggled for a long time to land a prestigious part. Everyone faces rejection. However, perseverance is the key. When you are not willing to give up, you could meet someone who will accept a "yes" instead of an answer.

You must continue to go out and making an effort. Do not surrender to self-defeat due to one rejection. A few rejections don't suggest that you will not be received by someone who is welcoming. If you give up and begin dwelling in fear you're at risk of missing this one unique opportunity.

The moment you stop working on your goals is when you are dying inside. Even if it seems like you are wasting your time or even futile it is impossible to abandon what is causing you to live your best your life. Your goals are what bring you the enthusiasm and motivation to keep going. Don't give up and never let up and go missing out on something that could transform your life to the best possible.

This is also true for the past rejections. It is possible that you have had a rejection in the past and are having a difficult time to overcome the experience. Rejections in the past may have diminished your self-confidence and self-esteem and caused a fearful feeling in your mind that you will not achieve success in a certain endeavor. However, the mistakes of the past do not have any impact on the future. It is possible to get a yes in the near future. Therefore, work hard to get over the past and not let the past mistakes keep you from achieving. What was once a rejection in the past could be a yes in the near future.

Find an alternative

Sometimes, you are stuck on a specific path. You're determined to reach the goal or perform things in a particular manner. The level of determination you display is actually a positive quality. It could mean that you have a great persistence. It is important not to abandon yourself and make a change in the event of a single disappointment. Thus, staying with your original strategy is a good idea.

Sometimes, you need to make changes to your way of life. Whatever you try, you're not in a position to conform to the norm of what you ought to be. A business concept or project that doesn't belong in a typical category may be a great idea but it could be difficult to promote to more mainstream people. It is possible that changing your strategy will result in more satisfaction.

It's not always easy to recognize that you need to make a change. You think you're in the right direction however, finding out that it's not. It can be a bit confusing to know how to reconsider and adjust your plans. Be aware that changing your plan and the direction you are taking does not necessarily mean giving up. It is possible to be stifled by pride from acknowledging that you're required to adopt a different strategy however, you shouldn't allow pride to stop you from making the right decisions about your personal life or business.

It's possible that all you have to do is modify the way you present. The manner you present your business plan or how you interact with a person will determine how you create a the first impression. We all know that poor first impressions can hurt you. Maybe there's something wrong with your proposal however, your presentation is unable to effectively sell your idea. Sometimes all you have to do is alter the presentation in order to make your proposition appear more appealing and positive. You are then likely to be more successful.

On contrary you might find that you need to alter the way you present your idea. It's not the presentation which is flawed, but rather you're giving people something they're uninterested in. It is necessary to rethink your approach and discover an alternative direction to put your idea. It is possible to alter your plan to take into account the local population or incorporate trends that are in fashion in the present to ensure it is more appealing to buyers. You might find that you have to take care of yourself, in particular the way you dress and how you conduct yourself to make yourself more attractive to other people.

Change the direction that you are going with your project could result in you finding another avenue to pursue your desires. If, for instance, you're trying to start modeling however you're overweight, you could either shed weight or attempt to do modeling that is larger. If you're looking to publish a novel that is genre-bending you should consider an indie publishing company , or self-publishing and selling through websites such as Smashwords as well as Amazon. You may discover that your business concept is fantastic, however, it isn't suitable for your particular region because it doesn't attract the demographics of your area and you must expand your company elsewhere or have an entirely different experience.

It is possible that the conventional methods don't work for you. So go a more unique route. If you're unable to get something to work try an alternative route or location. Don't give up. explore alternatives that could help you achieve your goals. Don't keep running into the wall and experience failure after defeat.

It is painful However, it is an indication of how to make improvements to your business or your self for success. Sometimes, rejection is the signal you require to figure out what you're supposed to do. Consider rejection as a useful instruction and point of reference rather than an act of punishment.

It's Just One Person's Opinion

There are billions around the world and billions of people around the world, focusing on the opinions of one individual is not wise. Don't let someone else tell you what you're like. You shouldn't base your perception about yourself on the opinions of one individual. Be aware that everyone's opinions differ and the opinions of one person may not necessarily reflect the views of all people.

Many times, people make the error of trying to blow someone's mind in their minds. They give too much weight to the opinion of one person. There are many people in your life who you'll want to impress. A parent, a boss an acquaintance, a potential client or lover The opinions of these people could be very important to you. However, sometimes, you're creating a risk for heartache by basing all of you happiness upon the viewpoint of a single individual. You are entitled to wish to impress somebody, but if aren't able to impress the person you are trying to impress then you're not insignificant. There's no excuse to let someone else's opinion ruin your confidence or dictate what you're worth.

If you're rejected by someone be aware that their judgment isn't necessarily a fact. If someone doesn't think you are good enough doesn't mean you're not adequate. Others may be interested in the qualities you offer and could consider you for a job. Rejection does not say any thing about you or what you've got to provide. It is something more to the individual who turned down you than it does about you.

Many rejections may make you doubt your worth. If many people don't think you're good enough, you might begin to question whether you're really good enough. It might appear as if the majority of votes are true. But , in reality, you're seeing a genuine majority vote. Since there millions of people living in the world, the views of a few people aren't all-encompassing.

When you hit a brick wall, and having to endure multiple rejections usually suggests that you are trying to create something fresh and exciting. Many people are afraid of expanding their perspectives. Your ideas and proposals could require them to make decisions that they are afraid to take. This doesn't mean you're not providing something that is valuable for the rest of humanity. The problem is that you're not reaching the appropriate persons with the exact vigor and creativity that you do. It is crucial not to be afraid to doubt yourself or quit because of the opinions of a few skeptics. Instead, you must continue to push forward. Try using different angles or to approach in different directions. There's likely to be to be a niche that is right for you but you need to locate it.

Use it as a way to Sell Yourself

Rejection can be the end of the road for certain people. However, don't view it as the end of an agreement. Instead, it could be the beginning of a new one. The word "no" is not always a guarantee. In fact, a no is an opportunity for you to show how much you desire something. If you are determined to get past the word"no" and begin selling yourself to transform the word "no" into "yes then you might win the respect of others around you particularly those who aren't embracing you. It will show that you're motivated and really need something. Also, you will become more desperate and will begin to convince yourself.

"The sale can't be started until someone doesn't say"no." The saying is well-known salesman's saying. If someone does not say yes it means you must make an effort to convince them to accept. It is now time to market yourself , your idea, or project with more enthusiasm.

A lot of people view no as a definitive answer. For those who want to succeed, they view no as a starting point in the process of negotiation. Instead of taking no as an answer, use the refusal as an encouragement to push yourself further. Allow rejection to motivate you instead of dragging you down.

The No Will Not Kill You

The most important part of being rejection-proof is to remind yourself that being rejected isn't an end in itself. In the course of evolution our brains are trained to make rejection as the most terrible possibility that could ever occur. In our modern world rejection by the herd doesn't cause you to die at the hands of a wild animal. It is possible to endure rejection and continue to move through the rejection process.

Consider the rejections you've experienced in your lifetime. Every one of them probably affected you in some way. A few may be so hurt that they felt as if they had reached the ending was near. Your self-esteem may be shattered and your confidence was smashed into smithereens. But you're still here. You survived those painful and painful rejections, but you came out without injury.

So, you'll be able to get through the next rejections also. It is likely to cause pain. It is not a good idea to lie and saying that rejection will not cause harm. If you're not accepted in any project it is likely that you will be able to survive. It's just a matter of picking off the pieces, and go ahead. Don't let the worry about something that will not actually cause you to die stop you from living your life fully and taking risks.

Chapter 3: Tips To Deal With Rejection With The Grace Of A Professional

In the last chapter, I spoke about the fact that you must be prepared for rejection in your life to accept that it's fact of life. If you are faced with rejection but you don't have to let it ruin your self-esteem or derail your work. Instead, you can develop the skills how to deal with the often-painful experience of rejection with ease. You can continue to live your career and avoid soaking in pain and anxiety with a few easy ways of coping.

Naturally, the first step to overcoming rejection successfully is changing the way you view rejection following the advice in Chapter 2. A more positive outlook on rejection will help you conquer your anxiety however, it will also help you manage rejection more effectively in the event that it happens. A positive attitude towards rejection can help you accept rejection and use it as an opportunity to make improvements to your business plan or even your craft. It is no longer a matter of viewing it as the final step on the line, instead it's the start of a new one. This perspective can help you deal with rejection in a way that's more conducive to solutions, and also better for your self-esteem.

Although you may have a positive outlook about rejection, it isn't easy. You can overcome the hurt by seeing rejection as an opportunity to grow, instead of a direct attack on your emotions or your self-esteem. You can put your energy and focus to finding new ways to be accepted instead of dwelling on the emotional hurt of being not accepted.

Create a learning Experience

The experience of being rejected is often a painful experience. However, you can lessen the pain caused by this experience by focusing on the positive aspects of the experience. Try to look on the positive side of the rejection in all of the positives it may offer you, not just the negatives.

You might be asking, "What could be positive about being rejected? I was just shot down! What can make me feel more content?"

The primary benefit of being rejected is that it gives you the chance to gain something. It is possible to learn about people around you, yourself and the work you do when face rejection. Rejection can indicate that something you've done wasn't good enough which can hurt. However, it could also give you a clue on how to improve your project enough in the future.

Some people are simply rude and will scold anyone without giving any kind of feedback. Some people are accommodating and provide constructive criticism in addition to their disapproval. If someone gives you constructive criticism, set your ego aside and take note. There might be something of significance to what they're telling you. You can make use of the constructive feedback to address any weaknesses or problems with your work.

Sometimes, listening to your instincts is all you need to do to make improvements to yourself. If you're a victim of rejection and you are convinced you know the reason, it is not a good idea to think that your fears are the reason for your disapproval. If you're certain that something that you feel uneasy about caused the rejection, then maybe your intuition tells you something important. Maybe you know there's something wrong, and your body is screaming to you to correct it. Be aware of your instincts and fix anything you think isn't up with your expectations as well as the standards set by your colleagues. In Chapter 2 I suggested not blame your fears for being rejected. Although this is a good advice, you should also look at your fears for suggestions on how you can enhance your own self-esteem. Sometimes, your fears offer clues to things that you would like to alter about yourself. If you make changes to those things you dislike concerning yourself, you might simply fix what's making others dislike you. This is for yourself , more so than others. If you are unable to alter how people view you but you will feel more confident. This will help you sell your products or concept with more enthusiasm. You'll be sure to appear more attractive and have greater success when you are more confident in yourself and display less anxiety.

If you're unable to determine the reason why you were not accepted and your instincts do not give any more insight into the issue If you are not sure, try to find out how you can succeed. Learn from other successful people go about their business. If, for instance, you find yourself constantly disqualified when writing proposals, take a look at the successful proposals of other professionals. It might help you gain insight on how to write proposals that can earn you a"yes. Another example is that you're trying to find an entry-level job in a particular area but are constantly rejected due to lack of prior experience in the field. You can compensate for the lack of experience by researching the field you're trying to enter and learning more about it so that you appear to be an appropriate candidate for the job you're seeking. Don't be afraid to research and discover all you can about the topic. Your understanding and subsequent confidence in the subject will help you stand out as an outstanding candidate.

Make use of rejection as a way to gain the most you can. Learn and study examples to acquire the knowledge and experience you require to become an ideal candidate for the job or for a collaboration. The rejection can be a signal to be more knowledgeable and well-prepared.

The rejection process can teach you difficult lessons on what people want and want. This can make you more attractive to potential buyers in the future. You will learn what is effective in the presentation and what is not. You are taught how to make your presentation more attractive. The process of resentment is essentially a love lesson on learning how to become more efficient and competitive in your work or creativity, as well as romantic relationships. You might find out that hanging around someone's neck isn't the best an effective way to portray yourself as a romantic companion. It is more effective to be sexy by offering them an alcohol drink is often better.

Take it as a loss for someone else.

If you're not accepted If you are rejected, it is helpful to recognize that it's the loss of someone else, and more so than your own. You must be sure that you can offer something valuable. If you are rejected by someone the person is the one to blame. You could move your brilliant ideas other and let another person profit from your collaboration.

Imagine how those who have rejected J.K. Rowling feel now. J.K. Rowling experienced hundreds of rejections when she wrote the first Harry Potter novel. She is now wealthier than Queen Elizabeth II of England and Harry Potter has become an internationally acclaimed franchise as well as an iconic brand. Everybody knows what the little wizard is, and nearly everyone is familiar with the book or watched the films. Agents who rejected J.K. Rowling really missed out when they chose not to represent her book.

People who don't like you right now are going to be left out. Your book or whatever it is you are trying to sell could become the next big thing. You are likely to earn an enormous fortune in the near future, just like anyone who is willing to give you a chance. People who turned you down are the ones who regret it in the near future, because they will miss out on millions of dollars and a lot of fame. They didn't believe in your abilities and, as a result they don't get to reach the highest levels in fame or fortune you.

A lot of people say the phrase "Your loss" in a flims attempt to gain false satisfaction. However, you don't have to get only false happiness from this notion. It is possible to truly feel better and be convinced of the worth of the services you offer the world by focusing on those who do not like them as fools who have missed out on something amazing. You can find someone who truly appreciates the value of what you provide. People who don't like your offer are making a major mistake!

Find New Motives to Live

You shouldn't depend all your happiness on one factor. In the event that you do so, you'll likely be disappointed and repeatedly. If you set out to achieve something only to be dismissed, you don't need to be feeling like you've failed your goal. There are many other opportunities that you can strive for.

It is important to never let go of an idea. However, if you think that your dream is impossible, you should not abandon your dream of living a life of excellence. Instead, you should begin to look for new goals and dreams. Don't give up on the lesser. Continue to strive towards excellence and attempting to achieve whatever you set your mind to. There's so much you can accomplish and to be around the world, you should not be a victim of the end of one project.

It is important to shift your attention away from the group or person that has rejected you. Instead, you should find new people who really want to collaborate with you or even be around you. Make sure you are focusing on new or old interests. Try to bring old ideas up to date. It's a good idea to turn your attention away from resentment and discover a new passion for living.

It could be the motivation you need to begin living an enjoyable life. If you don't like something, try it out, now you are able to test new things. You can shift your attention to more beneficial productive, profitable activities.

Your name is the Harbinger of your own destiny

There are two types in which you control the destiny of your life: both internal and external. External control refers to forces that are external to you that affect your happiness, your mood and thoughts. Internal forces are your attitudes and beliefs inside your mind which determine your future.

Rejection is typically an external force that may cause you to feel as if you've lost your grip. If you make contact with an individual, you are putting a part of your fate in the hands of them. If they do not accept you It can be like they're an immense, unstoppable force, similar to an apocalypse, destroying your life. It can feel as if you're being ruled by an outside force, and it can make you feel helpless and battered. It may be as if you're having a bad luck. If you quit focusing on the forces outside of yourself, you're able to doubt yourself since you can't realize the influence you have over your life.

It is essential to take the control back into your own hands. Don't think that you're worthless due to the external forces acted against you. In the end, you are the one who determines the future you decide to make. You have the option of letting go of the power that you possess, or return it. Invoking your own power will allow you to feel more confident and result in greater success in your life.

If someone doesn't like you, it doesn't mean you're in a position of powerlessness and dependent on other people. Perhaps you feel like that particularly in the business world where you depend on customers and investors to ensure your survival, but in reality you are the one in control. It is you who are who is offering clients something amazing. You have the ability to control that offer and begin to reject-proof yourself. It is possible to make your idea or product better by making a few adjustments. There are many avenues to explore.

Don't let go of the power to control your life and your destiny. Your internal forces have significant influence on your external forces. If you think positively and take an initiative you will start to take back control of your life and increase your chances of being successful.

Chapter 4: Get Rejected Less

It is impossible to stay away from rejection However, you can improve your appeal in order to feel less rejection. With just a few strategies, you can influence the external and internal forces around you to accept you instead of pushing you away. The odds of being disapproved or accepted remain fifty-fifty, in any situation However, you can turn the odds to your advantage by displaying confidence and making your presentation of yourself and your propositions with a more attractive manner.

Offer People Something They Would Like

Finding out what appeals to people is the key to making yourself more acceptable. Everyone is different and distinctive in their perception of what they want in other people. There aren't specific rules that work for all. It is essential to study the opinions of others and to learn about them quickly, so you can figure out the best way to reach them. Learn what kind of people they are interested in and customize your message to meet their preferences while keeping in mind their negatives.

It is important to be proficient in discerning people. If you see a gentleman who is well-dressed then it's appropriate to dress appropriately when you meet him. If a woman is wearing the scent of a particular floral it is likely that she is fond of that kind of scent. You can try to impress her with products that smell similar to her scent.

You can also get information about what people want by listening carefully as they talk. Do they talk about the fact they have an extended family? If yes, they most likely are looking for time with family or vacation time, financial stability, and money. Have they mentioned that they dislike being harassed at lunch? If yes, you should discover their lunch time and stay clear of texting or calling during lunch time.

Consider the culture one comes from. If they come from a different culture, you should research the mannerisms that are typical of their home country to determine what comes to appear the most attractive. For instance, looking tall could make you appear significant, which is typically attractive to people from America however not so much in other countries like Asian countries. Therefore, you should dress in heels that are high or other enhancing footwear when you meet someone who is American or a woman, and wear flats when you meet someone from the Asian background. Know the proper signs to use for respect and greetings and also. Some countries do not appreciate handsshakes that are firm and those who use their first language to communicate.

In business presentation is the most important thing. You must make your proposition appear in a manner that appeals to those who are in charge. Be sure your proposal provides them with the things you know they would like. Consider the industry you're planning to enter to ensure that you modify your presentation to fit their expectations. If you're in the field of creativity think about making your resume or presentation artistic. If you're entering the more conservative fields you can leave out the frills. Look over some examples of resumes or presentation examples for various professional fields to understand what you can do. The more attractive your proposal or presentation more likely it will be accepted.

Although everyone is unique however, there are some aspects that everyone can enjoy and. For example, dressing well and arriving punctual for a meeting for a job interview or meeting is an requirement that everybody shares. Fresh breath is also appreciated by everyone. If you're presenting something, it is important to keep it simple to avoid confusion. This can cause people to be offended particularly busy people. Some people are more relaxed than others, however it's not a good idea to make a fool of yourself. Always be courteous, respectful clean, neat and well-groomed when you meet people. You can boost your chances by attracting people with manners, cleanliness good appearance, and professional appearance.

You should be focusing on them, not You.

If you're trying to impress someone it is crucial to concentrate on how other people are benefited by working with you or even pursuing you. Don't make it about your personal preferences as well as how you want some thing. Many people do not and don't have the time to think about what you would like. Instead, you must make it appear as if everything is about them. Make sure you only offer advantages and make your offer enticing. Let them feel that when they accept you that they have purchased an entry ticket to paradise and solving all their issues.

Salespeople are experts in this. They are able to sell an item in a way that makes you feel as if it will enhance your life. Follow this example and make yourself a sale. Create yourself as the answer to the prayers of someone else. Don't be timid or shy since this isn't the right time to be doing it. Being confident and bold is essential to make others feel that you're worth being considered as a potential candidate.

Project Confidence

If you show confidence, you can inspire others to believe in yourself. Confidence makes you attractive and cause people to be more likely to accept what you're promoting.

There are numerous ways to look confident, even if you're not as confident in your own skin. One method is the way you present your self. When you meet anyone, maintain a confident posture, keeping an upright spine and chest up. Keep your eyes fixed to demonstrate that you don't have anything to hide, and nothing to be embarrassed of. Handshake your hands with firmness. Make it sound like you know the subject matter you're discussing. Avoid stuttering and stammering as well as using words that are placeholders such as "um," as these items can make you appear nervous. Make sure you use a more expansive language to demonstrate how knowledgeable that you really are. However, be sure to employ words that you understand the meanings of. Nothing will make you appear like a more foolish person than using words that are not appropriate in the contexts.

Maintaining your appearance is important. When you dress well it conveys that you value yourself and possess a good confidence in yourself. People who are rumpy look unattractive since they don't appear to be self-confident or feel good about their appearance. Try to to present yourself and look good. Look and dress for the occasion.

Talk as if the Deal is already in the Bag

One method for people to be influential is by making them feel as if the deal has already been made. This can make people feel as if they cannot turn you down. The idea of claiming that it's already sealed is a well-known sales technique. It creates pressure on customers to sign a contract because they feel that the deal is already in place and it is incorrect to refuse.

Beware of appearing alone

In a social test, an unidentified young man walked into an uninviting bar on his own and began chatting with women. He usually had pretty good luck with women at the bar he went to, where he was familiar with everybody, however when he tried to talk to women at this bar, there was no luck. Some of them even tossed drinks at his face.

Then, he returned to the bar but this time with a group of guys. They had a good time, drank beers, and laughed while playing darts. After just one hour of entering the bar the young man noticed that women were staring at him with awe. When he approached them and asked them questions, he realized that he got the luck of his life back.

This study shows how important it is to make it appear as if that you are loved by people around the world. If you appear to be loved by other people, you will create the impression that people are also a fan of you. This is due to the instinctual herd-like nature that people have. If you are a friend that you like, others desire to join in and become friends with you, as well. This shows everyone that you're liked and an integral part of the human population.

If you're seeking to stay out of the spotlight, make use of your network of friends and acquaintances to make yourself appear more appealing. Get endorsements. Make sure that people find you worthy of consideration. This will make them think it's an excellent idea to allow them to accept youtoo.

Be Consistent

Persistence is the key to success. You must be perseverant, even to the point that you are irritating. Utilize persistence to keep trying to achieve what you need. It is more likely that you succeed if you persist and don't give up.

Persisting shows how much you take pride in and how committed your commitment to something. If you demonstrate to that someone you care about it, they might be more likely to take an opportunity.

Persistence is the only way to stay ahead of the game. Don't quit and you don't get a chance to lose out. Continue to work until you get the chance.

You may also be able to pressure individuals into giving up and get off of them. But this kind of persistent behavior is risky. If you make someone angry excessively, you could lose their attention forever. It is important to remain persistent and assertive without appearing rude. Be sure to not contact you at inappropriate times or more than twice every day, for instance.

Feel emotionally disconnected

The emotional disconnect can result in negligence. However, it's not always a negative thing. In fact, it's recommended when you are making yourself vulnerable to rejection. Remove yourself emotionally from the aspects that are important to you, so that you look more confident and less overwhelmed by rejection.

Don't confuse emotional disconnection with being uncaring. Being emotionally distant from your job or other areas of your life doesn't mean you are not concerned. You should really care. However, you don't have to put all your joy into something. Also, you shouldn't depend on your life or your feeling of success on. Don't fall into the trap of thinking that one success that is a yes can solve all your issues and set you on the path to happiness forever.

A detached emotional state will allow you to appear confident instead of anxious. People are more likely to be confident than despair, and so emotional separation can benefit you over the long term. Be careful not to project any kind of desperation in order to win acceptance. The pressure of being desperate can cause you to look bad to those whom you're trying to convince. Do not think that an acceptance is an absolute requirement and a denial would be the end of the road. You have other areas in your life that you could take advantage of, as well as other options for action. This is how you be emotionally detached from your job and look more confident. Your confidence will be authentic If you have a backup alternative and don't rely completely on the approval of others.

There's a further advantage to removing yourself emotionally from the things. If you're emotionally detached the possibility of rejection is less likely to snuff your confidence. It's a fact of life, and you are able to accept it and go forward. Being emotionally detached will allow you to persevere and not to fall back into the pit of fear due to your wounded self-esteem.

Chapter 5: Diverse Kinds Of Rejection

Rejection can happen across all aspects of life. There are times when you will experience rejection, whether at work or in your personal life. It could happen at work, in school or even in your home with your family. The way that rejection affects you may differ depending on the situation, but it is always painful. You can discover different strategies to deal with rejection that are specifically to specific aspects of your life, but you must be able to reduce the impact.

Romantic Rejection

The impact of a romantic rejection is more than any other rejection. Breakups or hearing a "no" in the event that you want to ask someone out, or even propose to someone else can seriously damage confidence in yourself. There is many emotions, from frustration to anger to self-doubt, to sadness. It is often some time to recover from rejection of any sort.

Sometimes, a love rejection can be like experiencing withdrawal from a substance.

It is because the love hormones release such as testosterone, serotonin, and Oxytocin. These are all feel-good hormones and the abrupt stoppage of them could trigger an emotional withdrawal. MRIs have proven that the same area of brain that gets activated during withdrawal from cocaine also activates when a romantic relationship is rejected.

In addition, couples typically have shared memories. If you lose a person whom you've been with for a long time and you are unable to relive your memories. That's why breaking up could feel as if you've lost a portion of you. Two aspects of love can make a sudden breakup cause a lot of pain.

The emotional wounds that have been a part of your past can come back up after an unwelcome rejection, as you're brought back to the past. Past wounds can only increase the pain and ego is bruised.

It is essential to never let rejection from romantic partners discourage you from seeking out the true love of your life. If you've had numerous rejections over your life, it isn't a sign that you will be on your own until the end of time. Most people give up and get bitter after they have failed. In reality, the failure of relationships is usually not the fault of you. The words that are spoken about in romantic rejection typically speak more about the person who turned you down, not the person who rejected you. You can overcome the rejection of your romantic partner by recognizing that it's not entirely your fault, and you can seek out someone else who is who is better. If someone doesn't like you, consider it a sign the person you are with isn't right for you instead of believing that you're not worthy of being rejected.

If the breakup was evidently your fault, you can use it to learn from the experience. There are others out there that are worthy of your highest respect. It is possible to use your relationships that failed to teach you how to improve your relationship with your partner in the near future.

Also, you can make use of rejection to gain knowledge about your flirting techniques. If you are constantly turned down, think of it as to be a sign that your method is in need of improvement. Start developing your social skills, and work on your appearance.

If you're going through the aftermath of a breakup, take a look at the negative things that happened. Your entire relationship is likely filled with warning signs that indicated it wasn't meant to be. Consider your ex and the flaws that he or she has. It's highly unlikely that they are flawless. In time, you'll start to realize that you were not meant to be , and are do not match up perfectly. You will be free of guilt and self-doubt, and move through the process realizing that it wasn't your fault for being not accepted.

Social Rejection

The human instinctual need to be accepted as a member of the herd makes social rejection so challenging. Being rejected and feeling marginalized by others can stimulate the part of the brain which associate rejection with the possibility of death. It's not a great feeling.

There are many reasons to be rejected by society. You could be disregarded by society due to your choice of lifestyle. It is possible that you are socially awkward and not be able to communicate with others quickly. You might have a mental illness, disability or another issue which is not your fault and causes you to be a source of disdain and rejection from other people. There is a chance that you made mistakes in the previous life or been accused of committing a offense that has made those you love most berate you. Abiding by social norms in any way could cause you the subject of ridicule. If you're disregarded socially, it's not the fault of you. However, you have to endure constant discomfort and pain each time you are rejected by someone.

The pain of rejection from social circles could cause you to withdraw yourself to avoid feeling the pain. Fear takes over your life and feel lonely because you're afraid to continue putting yourself out in the world. Or, you might try to be someone you're not. You attempt to be accepted and discredit certain aspects of who you really are in order to make yourself appear acceptable in the eyes of society. Your efforts often fail and you end up becoming extremely unhappy and unsecure. The people who appreciate you frequently turned off by your fake appearance and you start to feel more rejection than you ever did when you were your own person.

Social rejection hurts. However, it's not a valid motive to turn to be someone you're not or to be a lonely person. It is not necessary to stop being social. It is just a matter of finding your passion. Finding your niche requires you to remain honest with yourself so that you will draw people who are similar to you.

It is also important to never alter your self-image. It is crucial to keep in mind that there is there is no one like you. You are your own. It's not a good idea to change your individuality by any means, and especially for others. People who are not yours are not worthy of your peace of mind or security. Most of the time, those who you value your opinions aren't worthy of your time or attention. They don't provide your with a monthly income, encourage you, or provide any other significance to your existence. So why do you need to devote all your time and energy into them? Get rid of them. Do not change yourself to fit in with them.

Creative Rejection

The one area that suffer the most discontent is with creative pursuits. If you're an artist or an inventor of any kind, then you've felt the pressure to invest all of your energy and your self-confidence into a task. You could spend hours, months and even years working on an amazing work. When you are done with your project you're convinced it's stunning and can't wait to showcase your work out to everyone else. But for some reason, others are not aware of the beauty and the depth the work. They don't understand or value your work. They may also appreciate work you believe isn't worthy of your time. The lack of respect other individuals show for your work could lead you to think about the worth of your work and it can also erode your self-esteem.

Art requires an amount of confidence and confidence and. It is essential to believe in your work in order to continue. You wouldn't put your energy and time into something you consider to be ugly and unworthy. So, you put the majority of your confidence in your work and consider your work worth acclaim. Rejection is usually a severe hit because it undermines your faith in your abilities and self-esteem.

The reality is that rejection and criticism in the art world is a given. The level of competition is also high. The esteem that of certain artists is due to relationships, not on the excellence of the art they create. This may be unfair, however it's the reality. Be aware of this whenever you feel the feeling of jealousy. Your work isn't poor. It's just not as widely praised.

Also, people have different tastes. It is likely that someone might not like your work. But that does not mean nobody else does. Some people may love your work. It is important to keep working and put yourself out there until you reach the people you want to reach. The more you showcase your artwork and the more people you will reach. Don't let a few critics cause you to feel that there is no one who will appreciate your work.

Concentrate more on the satisfaction with art and not on pleasing people. Your confidence will show on the way you present and your work. This can be a non-intentional way of creating fans for you.

Business Rejection

The process of obtaining grant money, investors customers or customers or even public attention for your company requires you to get yourself out in the open. This can lead to being rejected. The likelihood of rejection is high particularly in the business world, where the money is involved. People are very selective regarding where they invest their money, which is why they are very selective when it comes to investment and business transactions.

Marketing is the most important factor in overcome business-related rejection. It is essential to present your business plan in a manner that makes you seem worthy. Understanding the basics of marketing is essential to help you expand and market yourself within the world of business. Although the basics of marketing are beyond what is covered in this guide There are a few fundamental principles of marketing must be understood. First, you need to understand the demographics of your customers to determine the best way to appeal to those who are most likely to purchase your product. Second, you need to conduct market research and study the similarity of what other companies like yours are doing. In the end, you have to explain your findings to investors and utilize your research to develop a suitable marketing that appeals to your particular demographic.

Business failure is an inevitable element of business. However, it shouldn't affect your self-esteem. If people don't accept you, they could be missing an opportunity to earn a profit from your business. Be patient, and know that you are able to create your own progress. Trust in yourself and in your company.

Chapter 6: Overcoming Rejection

The Truth of Rejection

"The first story concerns connecting dots... Also you aren't able to connect the dots in the future but you can connect them backwards. You must therefore believe in the possibility that dots may connect in the future. You must trust something, your gut, destiny life, karma, or anything else."

-Steve Jobs, 2005

It can happen anywhere and for everyone. People experience rejection in their daily life, for example in love, school friendships, relationships, and even in family. Professional lives are also negatively affected when they are rejected, rejection of a proposition, a denial of job offer or an unsuccessful negotiation or partnership. There is no excuse for rejection, regardless of whether you're wealthy or not either old or young either gender well-known and significant or unnoticed and insignificant individuals are often rejected.

It's also hurtful. The feelings that accompany rejection can be characterized by sadness, loneliness, and even depression and anger. Things like anger, crying and even weakness are all part of the experience. Because as human beings human beings, we naturally need to feel accepted. Because each of us has the same limitations and limitations, we look for others to fill in the gaps of our own limitations. If we are rejected this is like our mental, physical and social are at risk. The threat is so real that it is difficult. That's why we react in the same way when we're not accepted. No matter how hard we try to cover up the hurt, our entire being is screaming for acceptance, even if it's not relief.

It is not always within our control, however our feelings, emotions and behavior are totally in our control. Now, you must not let it hinder your character, happiness and your destiny. It is not a reason to let rejection hinder you on your path. It will be there, but so is your courage, confidence and the drive to see your weight and persevere whenever rejection happens.

The following chapters will discuss the secrets of how to avoid rejection , but how to handle it correctly and overcome it triumphantly.

The transformation of a challenge into an opportunity

"I believe that you need faith in your destiny to succeed even though you will face lots of rejection, and it's not always straight and there are deviations, so take advantage of the journey."

-Michael York

The first step to overcome rejection is to change the way you view it into something positive. If others view rejection as negative, like a trap or a hurdle it is important to alter the way you view it. Instead, you should try an alternative view of rejection. Consider it as a positive thing or a way to get towards something more or a step towards something greater. Even when it's an absurd statement take it as a the rejection. Make use of the opportunity to consider alternatives, no matter how the differences are small.

Once you've been able to change your way of thinking, the next ways to overcome rejection become feasible. This is the primary step in achieving this achievement. I refer to it as an accomplishment since it isn't an easy road for you. It might not be as difficult as it was in the past however, it will cause pain. If you feel the pain that you feel, you may be discouraged or decide to give up on your efforts to conquer rejection. Before you dothat, think about what you'll regret, you may not become the person you're supposed to be. You might not be able to fulfil your dream or purpose or in a position to live the life you've always dreamed of or deserve to live. Get moving and continue to march to achieve this goal, not just to yourself, but also for your family members and friends who rely on you to overcome the challenges of rejection.

The Two Options: Short Term Relief and Long Term Resilience

"When there isn't a struggle, there isn't any force."

-Oprah Winfrey

The way to conquer rejection starts by changing it. The next steps are based on two fundamental principles that can help you overtake it. They are:

1. Relief for short-term issues

2. Long-term resilience

A short-term relief plan is the one that will help you to cope following being rejected. No matter how confident you are, nobody is protected from the immediate effects of rejection. These strategies will allow you to deal with those feelings and stop them from encroaching into your character and thoughts. By using these techniques to cope you can stop the feelings and provide with relief.

Long-term resilience is a different way to conquer rejection. It is designed to gradually increase your defenses and reduce the burden of rejection. These techniques for building resiliently will not only help your future self when rejection occurs, but they can also prepare you for rejection in advance. is right in the near future.

Take care to take action immediately.

Utilizing Positive and Self-talk

"Keep your eyes open to the sun and you will not see shadows"

-Helen Keller

Self-talk is a mental practice which helps to change the way you think. Through asking yourself questions, it allows yourself to come up with solutions that provide clarity or instructions for how to handle the situation. Self-talk can be an effective technique when used to overcome the fear of rejection.

Here are some of the questions you could ask yourself when you're fresh of a rejection

1. What is the reason for the refusal?

2. What lessons I can draw from this experience?

3. What options do you have following this denial?

4. Was I personally disapproved of or was it due to my own action or output?

5. How long will I be feeling this discomfort?

Answers to your queries might give you an abundance of information that you would not have If you are unable to stop and just focused on the hurt. You could, for instance, learn that the denial is not unjustified. There are solid reasons for why you weren't selected. It is possible to use this information to improve or further develop yourself when similar situations arise. If you've been rejected on the first choice, what do you feel about the next, third and the other possibilities that are waiting for you? They might prove to be more suitable alternatives, could mean you won't be accepted into if weren't rejected in the first in the first.

Many people, when disapproved of, believe they have been slapped in the face to themselves as well as their character. When you're able to remove yourself from your work it is possible to accept and move on following the rejection. If, for example, your proposal was rejected. Do not say or think, "I was denied." Instead, state it precisely as it is "The proposal was not approved." In this way,, you can distinguish yourself from the result. Instead of wasting your energy as well as your time, you could return to the original idea and figure out ways to modify it or look for those who are willing to accept it.

The moment you receive the rejection, regardless of whether you've got resilience or the coping skills to face it, the most likely you'll feel hurt or you will feel irritated. Instead of trying to ignore the feeling, it's crucial to allow yourself the time to feel it. Accepting the feelings is healthy as it allows you to process and comprehend the feeling. Refraining from these feelings will only stop your from learning from your feelings and anticipating the reactions whenever rejection occurs again. But, ensure that you establish an appropriate amount of time to experience these emotions. If you are unable to carry out your daily duties due to these feelings and you are unable to do so, then take a step back and continue to move ahead.

If you can honestly answer these questions, then you will be able to tackle rejection in the right and most effective method. Self-talk comes from a different method to overcome rejection, which is known as positive thinking.

Positivity is an intentional choice that you make to concentrate on the positive aspects of whatever circumstances you might face and simultaneously looking forward to the same good fortune for your future circumstances. You can use the same strategies to overcome the fear of rejection.

You can, for instance, opt to get rid of any negative associations you may have in relation to rejections and substitute them for positive ideas and thoughts. You can also continue to change thoughts concerning rejections. Your thoughts can be formulated into something objective and instructive instead of emotional and personal.

Action: Create the list of questions like the ones provided within this article. Recall what was the latest or painful rejection. Utilize the experience to answer the questions mentioned above. It is also possible to write the answers when you've got them. Utilize both lists to review the rejection before beginning with a positive attitude towards rejection.

Looking for and receiving social support

"Dearer do those regard us for being unworthy, because they bring another life to us; they create a paradise before us, wherein we have never imagined, and thus provide to us with new power sources from the depths of the soul, and encourage us to try fresh and untried actions."

-Ralph Waldo Emerson

Catharsis can be described as a way to refer to the expression of your emotions to an individual or something else and, it helps to reduce the effect or even relieve from similar feelings. You can experience emotional release when you are rejected by sharing them with someone you be confident in.

A person who is willing to be genuinely listening to you can provide you with an opportunlty to let go of your feelings of anger, frustration, and so on but will also give you an objective perspective regarding the rejection. They are your true friendswho can inspire you and also point out why you were rejected.

Social support can also be beneficial in helping you overcome the feeling of being rejected. They can assist you in going through the process and keep you from sinking into these feelings. However ensure that you're cautious in choosing people with whom you'll be sharing your story.

Another thing to remember when seeking social support is to refrain from posting your thoughts on social media. It's a grey space when you are expecting support because it's open to the public , and you could receive feedback or feedback that can hurt or cause more harm for you. If you share an item on Internet there is a good chance that it will remain there for a long time and could only bring back the disappointment instead of helping you go on with your life.

At the final point, so you're capable of receiving assistance from trustworthy people and have a trusted support system, it serves the function of the support system. If it's done in person or online, it proves that having someone to share your feelings will surely help relieve the feelings of rejection that are negative.

Step: Choose from your most trusted friends whom you will call when you experience rejection. Make a list that includes at least two or three of your closest friends who possess this trait. From this list, create an agreement to be supportive of one another and to keep each other's side in case the moment of rejection arrives. It is possible to create this pact by using any method of communication you feel comfortable with, however the goal is to cement this support and to be confident that you'll have other's back when knocking at a door and are met with rejection. This will become the ultimate definition of a system of support.

By using Bathing, Breathing, and Other Physical Relievers

"I am crying at my loss over something that I did not have. It's ridiculous. It's ridiculous to be mourning something that was never."

-- E.L. James

Sometimes, psychological relief through positive thoughts and self-talk, or social relief through the support of trusted friends may just not suffice to relieve your feeling of being rejected. Sometimes, you need to look for physical relief.

Try breathing exercises that can lower the heart rate and reduce the blood pressure. This can create a relaxing and soothing effect to an otherwise stressful experience. Sitting straight and closing your eyes and taking deep breaths, you can take deep breaths. Inhale through your nose , then exhale out of your mouth. While you inhale by your nostrils, visualize the white light coming in and rest your mind on the phrase, "positivity in." While exhaling your mouth, visualize taking out all the negative thoughts and stress that life brings, and resting on the words "toxicity out." Do this slowly and repeat this for up to five minutes.

A warm beverage can help offset the feeling of cold following a rejection. You can sip a hot cup of tea or take yourself a bath. The warmth soothes and can help to calm the thoughts running around your head.

While it's a temporary solution, focusing on other activities can help you to cope with the rejection. If you take a trip to do something completely different and isn't related to the reason for rejection, you will be able to distract yourself from the issue. You can leave the office, go on the road, or play your preferred sport. You can begin the book you've been wanting to read, or buy something you've always desired. These exciting and fresh experiences can not just shift your focus away from rejection, but also help you see that there are other aspects in your life that aren't the rejection.

Action: If you are feeling anxiety or stress that causes your heart rate to increase Utilize the breathing technique previously mentioned. Test the effectiveness it has on you. If it's effective, try frequently until it's instinctual response when you experience similar emotions. If it's not a method you like, you should research other breathing exercises on the internet and give them a go. There's no single right method to perform something. The breathing exercises mentioned as a doorway, opening your eyes to new perspectives, and the chance to overcome the negative impulses when rejection hits.

Practicing Introspection

Develop Your Vision, Passion and purpose

"Rejection is simply an opportunity to redirect your attention; a change in your course."

- Bryant McGill

The development of resilience is an vital step in getting over rejection. It acts as a buffer from being impacted by the rejection. If you can define your goal, vision or goal, then you're better placed to guide yourself when you face rejection. The first step is to create your vision or mission.

Finding your passion in life is a continuous task. But, one of the most effective ways to finding your purpose is by following your passion. The pursuits, the business or career job you enjoy doing or are the most enthusiastic about tend to be the reason for your life. Take a moment to reflect on the things you love about. Note it down. If you're still feeling a bit anxious, return to the breathing exercise you did before and repeat it at a slow pace for five minutes. After that, think about, "What am I really interested in? What am I passionate about that helps me become more of a person? What is it that I do that gives me the feeling that the clock never stops?" Write it all down. This will provide you with some idea about what you think your goal in life could be. Important to keep in mind is that the reason you are here could shift. Do not stress about it. It's simply an outline for your choices. Enjoy your goal and ensure it is enjoyable whenever you consider it. The goal you set will not be flawless. It will be refined over time. Relax!

Once you've got an inkling of the things your goal could be, it's now time to formulate your vision. Vision is more than just a notion It is something you can define, measure and define a period of time and even see and feel. Make use of this vision of yourself to figure out the place you'd like to be in the near and long future. It could be called your future, dream or even a goal. Whatever you decide to refer to it as, you can use it as a lighthouse when you guide yourself through your day-to-day life. As you will see, your mission and vision will set the path for your life, and the goal is more specific , which allows you to better concentrate on what is fulfilling instead of constantly getting distracted by things you consider to be urgent distractions. If you are able to stay focused on the purpose, you'll be able to accept failures as part of the process.

For instance, if you're aiming to land the dream job you've always wanted, make use of the same goal whenever you experience rejections. If you have been denied, keep your eyes on your final goal. Are you still in the position you want to be in the works? Sure, but it's not only within that particular business. Are there other options? It is only possible to find out by resuming your search.

Action: Create your vision by using an SMART approach. The acronym stands for specific, measurable, achievable pertinent and time-bound. Instead of stating your dream job, you should make it smart. Make it clear by stating that you are an executive. Consider it as earning a salary in the six figures. It is important to ensure that it is achievable by examining your qualifications and experience. Make sure your vision is current and relevant. Set a date for it. For example, 10 , 20 or even 30 years from today. Remember how your plan will continue growing.

Being able to identify yourself using the Johari Window

"A man is merely the result of his thoughts What he thinks will become."

-- Mahatma Gandhi

Self is known to Self, but not to Self

It is known to other

Not widely known to the public.

One of the most effective methods to increase your resilience is to figure out who you are. If you are aware of what you can accomplish and also what you're not, you're much better placed assess and adapt yourself when rejection comes. You can draw on your strengths to help you get through rejection and tackle your weaknesses prior to them weighing you down. Johari Window Johari Window is an effective assessment tool that lets you know what you are aware of about your own self.

While it's done with your fellow students to aid you in making comprehensive assessments You can also apply it to assess yourself.

It is basically a table that has two columns and two rows, creating four boxes. First column marked as "known to self" while the second column is not identified to oneself. One row has the label as 'known to others' while the final row is labeled 'not not known by others.'

The upper left-hand corner Consider what you've heard about yourself and , at the same time other people know about you as well. Make adjustments to the size of this box to show your true public image. In the upper right corner Ask yourself: what about you are people aware of however you are not aware. Repeat this exercise for the rest of the boxes.

When you've finished altering the lines of the boxes within your window, you are able to estimate roughly how much you actually are aware of about you. The more wide the first column is , the more you are aware of yourself. If the first column is slim it could mean you have plenty of questions to ask about your self.

No matter what instrument you employ regardless of the tool you use, it is essential to be aware of your own capabilities and the resources available to you.

Action Take action: If the column is too narrow, seek for the assistance of your family and acquaintances in your quest for self-discovery. Ask them to judge your honesty as best they are able. Respect their opinion and listen to them. Make use of their advice to help you to help you overcome rejection.

Here's a list of useful adjectives you and your friends could make use of to evaluate yourself:

Additionally This website also offers an impressive set of questions for every aspect of your life, which will increase your awareness of yourself (I personally do not have a connection to this website in particular however, it has added tremendous value to my experience when I had a lot of anxiety and felt very unsecure after graduation).

Identifying the Roots of Rejection

"A rejection is only a vital step to pursue success."

- Bo Bennett

Being aware of the location and date of the battle enhances your chances of winning. The same applies to the battle against rejection, and as with all things, you need to be hopeful for the best even though you prepare for the most difficult.

Create a contingency plan for the case of rejection. What are you going to do? Where are you going? Who do you talk to? What are your options for responding? If you've got this plan you'll be more prepared to handle the situation. This will stop your from making a mistake you'll regret later on or to do something which may make you look embarrassing at the time of rejection.

You could also enhance your knowledge by recalling instances in which you were disqualified. Was it because you were unprepared or pressured to time? Was there tension within the relationship that resulted with rejection? Did your gut told you to be prepared for rejection? If you can recall these events and identify a pattern. If these issues come up again, it is possible that rejection will come knocking. If you can anticipate it, you'll be more prepared. The better prepared you are and the more efficiently you are able to deal with rejection and overcome it.

Then try to think of at least three occasions during your life that caused you to be rejected. were dismissed. Find a pattern or a connection in these three. Make use of the list to identify warning signs to be aware of. For instance, you'll always be rejected if you approach someone who is in an awkward or shy state. The next time you approach someone make sure you are confident and assertive, and then see whether there have been any some changes. If you're accepted, you've found a way utilize past failures for your benefit. You can read and watch about this easy exercise to better understand your physiology in both empowering and disempowering situations.

Building confidence

Celebrate Your Strengths

"I do not have an enviable level of self-confidence, however I am aware of the blessing I've received from God and try to give it to the most people I can."

-Andrea Bocelli

Building confidence prior to and regaining confidence after rejection is another way to build the ability to overcome. Every person has a unique ability, talent, or talent. Whatever it is, it could be the sciences and sports, the writing, arts and creating, planning, or any other area there is something you excel at and should feel proud about. Although you might have some weaknesses however, it is essential to turn your attention away from them.

Strengths and , more importantly, properly acknowledging and recognizing that they exist can help you to create defenses against the negativity of feeling rejected. Believe in your own abilities and the resources available to you can help you over the fear of the fear of rejection. Utilize these strengths to help yourself when faced with rejection. Take pride in your achievements and achievements. A single failure is nothing to the many strengths, achievements as well as friends, accomplishments, and other good things that happen in your life.

Be aware that there is a line that separates being confident and arrogant. Make sure you build your confidence; often, your accomplishments are attributed not only to you, but also to those who helped your efforts.

Action: Create an assessment that reflects your best qualities. Begin by making the list of adjectives that best describe your currently. Some of your qualities will be obvious to those who are not you. It is possible to have them write their qualities for you. A few examples include: kind, artistic unique, individual active, perceptive, flexible, cheerful, loving beautiful, responsible imaginative as well as supportive, confident and reliable. You could use your 3-4 people with whom you have decided to be supportive of when you are rejected and ask them to give their opinions on your strengths. It will help you build relationships with them. You can determine their strengths.

Addressing Your Challenges

"Our biggest weakness is abandoning. The best way to achieve success is to give it a go another time."

-Thomas Edison

Although it is a feat of confidence to identify the strengths you have, it is a matter of the courage to write down your weaknesses. To be able to accurately assess your requirements against rejection you should also be ready to confront your obstacles. This will provide you with an understanding of the risks that could lead to the negative emotions or failures to deal with rejection.

Be aware that listing your struggles is not intended to make you feel sad, but rather to accept them as a part of who you are. Certain challenges are able to overcome, however, there are others that already form part of your persona. They are a present, instead of falling due to them, understanding that they exist will enable you to steer clear of or bypass them.

There are bound to be obstacles , however instead of allowing them to derail you, try picking yourself up each time. Similar to Edison He didn't let the difficulties from more than 10,000 errors stop him from inventing the bulb that lights up. He made use of his mistakes and obstacles to gain knowledge until he achieved the point of success. You are able to do the same yourself. Use your difficulties for your benefit. Utilize the lessons learned from the mistakes that you make due to your life's challenges as a means to achieve success.

In the same manner that you listed your strengths it's time to write down your weaknesses. This could also require the assistance of your trusted family members in creating an accurate description of your skills.

Building a Confident Attitude

"The soul inside me is something that no one will be able to degrade."

-Frederick Douglass

Rejection can affect confidence in yourself, but the reverse is also the case. Self-confidence can reduce the impact of rejection. A more confident and positive attitude is the culmination of acknowledging your strengths and confronting the challenges you face.

Once you've completed your an evaluation of your own strengths and limitations and weaknesses, you can begin to expand your sources of confidence by involving your friends, family and loved ones. Keep them close They will be by your side regardless of what. They'll be aware of when to help and when to grant you some space.

If you've got a support group to help you and support you, it is also important to expect to meet a few people whom you encounter on your journey that might not be supportive. They could constantly be against your efforts; they may challenge your resilience or your level of resilience. They are not under your control and it's not in your power to alter them to benefit you. The best defense from them comes with a strong and consistent approach.

Action: List down the people who, circumstances or situations can be the main cause of your disapproval. Utilize empathy to determine the causes behind their disapproval of you. If it's within your control, then you have the power to alter their perceptions and opinions about you. If it's out of your control, then you should decide not to be worried or to be irritated by them. Accept them for what they are and count on yourself and your community to help you overcome the rejection from the people who are causing you to suffer.

Tony Robbins says that the value of your responses lies on the nature of your inquiries. Two extremely effective questions you can ask during this exercise are "What's amusing in the situation?" and "What's beautiful about this?" It might be beneficial to return to the breathing exercises prior to exercising those muscles that allow you to empathize. This will help you to get into an improved state of mind and you'll be able to access greater sources within yourself to get better answers. Try it out and be amazed by the positive results you can generate.

Chapter 7: Dating And Relationships

Everyone has the inherent desire to be part of something and feel a sense of belonging. This desire is most satisfied when you're capable of creating, developing and maintain relationships with someone else, whether it's you are a girlfriend, boyfriend spouse, partner, or even a lifelong friend. A special person in your life could be among the most satisfying experiences you could ever have. You've got someone you can count on, to show your love , and in some cases they even have a purpose in life.

However the rejection of these relationships could be an extremely difficult feelings that one could experience most likely throughout their lifetime. There are many kinds of relationships that are rejected. It could be someone looking to be accepted by someone who he loves, but being not accepted. It could happen during an affair and, due to a reason or another the relationship ends or you fall apart. There are many scenarios to consider and will each have various reactions to the rejection. Here are some suggestions to overcome rejection whenever they occur to you:

* Be aware of that there are stages in rejection as a result of loss

Beware of being a victim

Examine your partner's motives

* Be civil

* Try it again

The feeling of being rejected by your partner is exactly like losing because you're actually losing the person you cherish. If this happens, it's normal to experience phases that are similar to those who have lost a loved ones, whether through separation, distance or death, among other reasons. The stages and the emotions that you are likely to be confronted with are denial, anger bargaining, depression and acceptance.

In the stage of denial it is impossible to believe that you have been rejected. Once you start to recognize that rejection is taking place or has already occurred, you'll be angry toward your partner, yourself or others. To save the relationship, you'll start to bargain, and you'll declare that you are ready to let go or accept certain requirements. The feeling of loneliness or sadness comes when you're unable to restore the relationship and start to be down. In your introspection, you start to reflect, heal, and finally take the rejection as a sign of acceptance or over come the feeling of rejection.

Note that these stages aren't necessarily chronological in their nature. According to your personality, you could skip the stage you are in and be accepted faster than other people. You may also combine two stages and experience a variety of emotions simultaneously. There isn't any time frame for these stages. Some can traverse the process in just a couple of months, while others will require several years. Many may not be able to recover from rejection. Knowing these stages can make you more prepared to handle these feelings. It will be clear that with time it will be a healing process.

A frequent reactions when you are you are rejected by your partner is feeling like victimized. You may feel that there's an issue, that something unfair happened to you, or it's something you are not worthy of. This is a normal emotions to experience particularly in the initial days following the rejection. But, these feelings can become risky when they are experienced for a long time. If you're not in a position to lead the normal life due to these emotions, you require professional assistance to overcome the issue.

Although it might appear to be the most important thing on your head, you should look at the reasons for your rejection. Examine the reasons, and if you believe them to be true you can use them to build your social skills as well as other aspects. Sometimes, your ex-partner may not always be able to provide the reason for their behavior, and when it happens, do not put words into his mouth. Avoid trying to analyze too much and place into the wrong assumptions.

It might be difficult at first , but you will be able to move on faster in the event that you decide to be friendly with your ex. If you are unable to distance yourself from them, the more likelihood that you will be able to hold on to feelings of anger, displeasure or any other negative emotions. Instead, decide to be more positive by reestablishing your relationship with them in a non-romantic however, still a friendly and respectful manner.

The most effective method to get over the rejection of an affair is not to just leave but to also attempt again. If you're ready, you can you can open your mind for the chance of finding love. Don't let past experiences stopping you from looking for new relationships, and maybe even finding that you like the most. you. Rejection in relationships can be overcome with an outcome of learning more about yourself, so that you can improve yourself for the next one.

Family

One of the supposed pillars of love, unconditional care and respect is family. It is that a child develops as a teenager, where a teenager develops his identity, and adults become parents. The family environment is what makes all this development possible due to the strength of unconditional acceptance of the family members. Family is a person's sanctuary it is the only place they feel they belong, a place where they feel safe regardless of what, and the final place where the possibility of rejection is a reality.

The truth is that family relationships are one of the most common situations in which people can be a victim of rejection. From childhood to until adulthood, it is possible to experience rejection. The issue of handling rejection from within the family is due to two aspects. One is the shock or surprise which is experienced from those unaware of the existence of the family's rejection.

Another reason is that when rejection occurs is a common occurrence in the family , especially in the early years of the person who is rejected it is common for people to either perpetuate the rejection, or be a victim of it over time. Studies have proven this. For instance, a child who is rejected by their parents tends to be a negative influence on their children once the parents become themselves. If a wife is divorced from her husband, it is common for women to be skeptical and cautious of potential partners due to the past experiences. Other scenarios indicate an unending cycle of being rejected.

The most frequent instances where rejection can occur include:

* A child who is rejected by an adult, such as abandonment

* A parent who is rejected by the child, for example rebellion

* Siblings who are siblings to one another for example, as is the case with rivalries that result from rivalry

* A parent of an adult, like separation or divorce

* A family unit refusing to accept an individual or a group, like being excluded

Whatever the individual who are involved, the rejection within families can be overcome by these steps.

* Recognizing the signals of rejection

* Verbalization of the feeling rejection

* Identifying the cause

Accepting the reality

1. Resolution for the reject

* Disconnect if required

* Creation of a family

Recognizing signs of rejection requires knowing the signals of rejection. Note that rejection may occur in various ways and can be expressed in different ways. Actually, the majority of rejection within the family doesn't begin with a verbalized denial. Before you get the message "No" or "I don't want to hear from you," you will receive non-verbal messages that could be a sign of not just imminent rejection, but also currently being disapproved of.

For instance, if you're a wife, and you notice the husband slowly getting physically distant from you This could indicate an indication of rejection. Sometimes, rejection is so subtle or subtle that it's often misinterpreted for something other than rejection. If, for instance, you're a child who receives only financial assistance from your parents but receive very the least amount of attention from them or any emotional reaction These distances could be interpreted as rejection. It is important to look out for either sudden or gradual change in the behavior of your family members to gauge the possibility of rejection.

If you are able to make these assumptions then the next step to check is the validity of these assumptions or not. Don't let your assumptions remain in that state, whether they are proven or not. It is impossible to live your life based on these thoughts. Therefore, you should express your feelings in writing. Make the effort to speak to your family member for clarification directly. Do not start your answer with a sarcastic stance Do not inquire "Why do you feel that I am being rejected by you?" Instead, you could express your feelings such as, "I am feeling rejected by the way you are acting current situation If I'm not wrong, Please let me know." It is possible to find that there isn't any rejection to be overcome.

If you do find that there is rejection it is important to allow yourself the time to consider the root of the problem. Was it something you did? Did it happen because a relative did? Does it happen in or outside of the family? Are you able to change it? can alter? Perhaps your family members can be changed? The most important thing in this case is to keep the communications lines open. In lieu of letting this thought grow in your head by tucking it away in your mind, let it come out into the open. In this way, healing begin.

When you're trying to determine the root of the problem You must acknowledge the situation. Nothing positive can come from denial. The sooner you acknowledge that you have been rejected by a person in your family, the faster can you begin to take action to overcome the issue. Denial can take many kinds; there are instances when you're hiding from yourself and not even realizing that you are. For instance, you could continue to make excuses for your family's actions in order to hide the fact that you are gaining distance among you and your family members.

Once you've gone through these steps, you are able to begin to resolve the reasons for the rejection. You may approach them, or ask for forgiveness, or find other solutions that addresses the primary reasons for rejection at the beginning. Start by using the methods that are shared with you in the first chapter of this guide to overcome the feeling of rejection. For instance, you could think positive thoughts to help you deal with your circumstances. It is also possible to ask for help from others, like other relatives of yours to aid you through the process.

However, you have to acknowledge that there are circumstances where the reason for the rejection is not solvable. In order to overcome rejection, you must allow the situation to run its course. As an example, you might require separating yourself from family members and your home for a time. Find a new accommodation, take a trip to a friend or an acquaintance. Allow your family and you time to consider your thoughts. The process of overcoming rejection might not be achieved overnight, but perhaps within just a few weeks, can sit alone and think about the various options.

Your family doesn't define you, but only you are able to prove and maintain your self-worth. Even if your spouse or family members don't like you The first person to be able to accept you is yourself. If you've considered all possibilities and attempted everything in your power however you still aren't accepted If you are still not accepted, it could be the time to say goodbye to your family member who rebuffed you. Get the support of your most trusted close family members or your friends. Keep in mind that you are the only person who can make decisions for yourself. If the situation is not resolved and you are resentful by your family members The only thing left to complete is to establish your own family.

Social Groups

Social groups are another type of relationship type in which rejection is possible. Although rejection from these groups can not create the same level of stress, anxiety or devastation as other relationships, these types of relationships have a different negative effect on the person. For instance, important opportunities or networks are lost if access to these networks is not provided. The privileges or perks you've always wanted might not be available.

There are many different scenarios that fall within this category:

* Rejection from a club or social association

* Sororities and fraternities and similar groups

* Professional associations

If these rejections happen and you are unable to overcome it, try one of these strategies to get over it:

* Learn

* Retry

* Look for sponsors

* Get moving

The majority of these social networks have a strict policy to allow admission. If you are experiencing the initial feelings of emotion following the rejection, make sure to apply the strategies described in Part 1. For instance, if the country club you belong to refuses membership, you must to take the lessons learned from the rejection. Find out the reason for the rejection.

Was it because you could not meet a specific standard? Do you have any way that you could do to achieve this standard? What are the other members' behavior? What can you do to change? Find out the fundamentals and beliefs that the group holds. Find out ways you can be a part of these ideals to more easily fit in with their group.

If you've done your research and gained knowledge from your experiences then the following step is to do it again. Find out how the teams will permit an opportunity to try again or for an opportunity to try again. If you know the information, take them and apply these. Make the most of your past experiences of rejection to push you to your success in this endeavor. Keep in mind that rejection does not necessarily be the end of your quest toward acceptance, it could be an opportunity to try something new.

One of the primary aspects that will help you not just overcome, but possibly overcome social rejection is by contacting sponsors. Sometimes, even with thorough study and utilizing previous experiences, the help of a member in the group will improve your chances of being accepted. Knowing who's in the group, and having access to the information only accessible to members, and other suggestions that could assist you in getting into the group and be successful on the second attempt can be obtained from sponsors. If you you're successful in convincing this sponsor to publicly declare their endorsement of your efforts, their public endorsement can go a long way.

There are instances when any effort you put into it will not make you a member of the group you have chosen. In these instances it is best to search for alternative options to your group. Choose a different group that will provide the same or near to the same benefits your chosen group could provide. Don't let the disapproval of this group stop you from the possibility of join another. You may think as if you're picking the wrong option, but don't let this idea rule your mind. It won't bring you anything good rather, adopt an optimistic outlook and think that this group could be hesitant to accept you as the better group is more suitable for you.

Before you start on this path of doing all you can to be a part of an organization, it is essential to first conduct your own personal review. Do you require any adjustments in any way? Do you need to modify your behavior to meet their standards? First of all is it necessary to be part of this particular group? Sometimes , while trying to be accepted by the groups you join, it is easy to lose sight of who you are. You are forced to give up too your own self. You could also exhaust all of your resources in the effort to find acceptance. You must decide with a sense of urgency to strike a balance between your choice of trying for acceptance or getting over your rejection by moving forward.

College

The college experience is an era for the majority of people. Being accepted into one's college brings immense happiness and joy to the students who have applied. Acceptance also provides them with a an elation and guidance for the future. But, the same amount of satisfaction that comes when someone is accepted could also be the feeling of fear and anxiety when one is disqualified. The young adult with his entire life ahead of him, to be interrupted with a rejection letter from a school can create anxiety.

The process of dealing with rejections from the colleges you've applied to can be handled by using different strategies that increase your understanding of the reason for rejection or the possibility to request reconsideration. There are a variety of methods to use:

* Understanding college profile information

* Expansion of options

* Resolving humiliation

* Allowing it to let it run its course

If an applicant is rejected there are a variety of factors that contributed to the rejection, and some of these factors do not directly reflect the personality of the candidate. Each college has its own individuality that affects their decision about whether to accept or deny applicants.

A university, for instance, that is known for its high standards for students who excel and its students who are active is likely to favor one student over one who is more relaxed. A school that is focused on science will select an applicant over one that seeks people who are passionate about the arts. So, if you're not accepted to an institution this does not mean you didn't succeed but you're a better fit in another place.

This means you'll need to broaden your choices. A college's rejection doesn't necessarily mean you will be rejected from all the other colleges there. Be more willing to consider other institutions of higher education, and having more than one choice for your college experience, choose three, five or more. Pick Ivy League institutions, state and community colleges. If you do not pass one of them, you have three more to choose from.

One of the primary concerns of those who are not accepted is peer pressure or shame that comes with being not accepted. Students often submit their applications in groups as do other students. If one student fails then the entire group will realize that he not succeeded. Find the courage to forget the shame that you feel and instead use them to increase your efforts in finding the perfect college for you.

While you are able to prepare yourself for rejection but there will always be a mild or extreme anxiety that comes with when you get the depressing rejection letter. If you receive a rejection letter, it will be normal to experience these feelings, but don't put them off. Instead, let them flow through your body and let the emotions flow. It is normal to feel sad scared, anxious or worried, but if you've allowed you to experience these feelings feelings and let others know about it like your family or friends , you will feel much more relaxed than if you were to keep it to yourself.

Another option you could consider in order to avoid rejection on colleges is to look at other alternatives that aren't related to the traditional college. College is a crucial aspect of establishing your professional career, but it's not the only avenue open to you. Setting up a company on your own, developing your interests and other opportunities are still open for those who haven't completed their college degree. Rejection from colleges isn't an end in itself however it could be a opportunity for you to open a door.

Chapter 8: Preparing For No

The process of overcoming rejection doesn't just require methods that can be applied after rejection has taken place. In order to beat rejection, you must to be prepared before it happens. The preparation in case of "No" is about making plans in the event of being not accepted. The more you prepare for the possibility of rejection, the better will be able to overcome it if it happens.

Planning for rejection can include planning contingencies and plans Bs and other alternatives to aid you in recovering after rejection does occur. If you have these plans in available, the sting of rejection is less brutal. If you're a student who is looking to attend the perfect college, don't place all your eggs, or for that matter, college applications in one basket. You must cover all the colleges you can. In this way, if you're not accepted by one college there are several other colleges waiting to take you in.

If you're looking to set a goal for sales, then you must be prepared for all possible situations. Look for more than one prospective client or customer. If you're dating and are looking for a partner, then be available to meet the many people you can instead of searching for the perfect person. If you'd like to belong to a social club look for other groups that offer them the exact benefits you are looking for.

You can also simulate the scene in which you're disqualified. What feelings will you experience? What lifestyle changes will take place? What are your immediate reaction? What are the resources you will lose? If you consider the possibilities, you will be able to prepare yourself to ensure that you do not get awed by the situation following the rejection. If you have these plans , and plan for the scenarios you'll be less worried about the event. If you know you're well-prepared, you'll feel relaxed in these situations which will increase the likelihood of success.

Note that planning ahead isn't a ensure that you won't receive a no. But planning will more than just prepare you for rejection. Rather, it gives you a degree of calm that will ease the anxiety.

Be prepared for the Yes

While it is crucial to plan in the event of a catastrophe, it is important to remain positive. This is when the notion of trying to fake it until you get it is practical. The idea is that you must imagine yourself in the moment of triumph. The same questions you ask yourself when making plans for the No, like what you would look , how you conduct yourself, how you communicate, and more are a good idea to ask.

Then, begin acting upon these cues that you have visualized. Dress up as like an individual who is loved instead of those who are not accepted. Continue to behave in as to appear like you're pretending that you already have been accepted. The self you will be in the future eventually merge with your current self. You'll realize that you're not doing anything or acting like it, but you are actually the person you're accepted.

If you are confident in your attitude of being accepted from as little as your manner of speaking, behave and speak to the thoughts you are thinking and the choices made, every one the above will reflect in your actions. People who you wish to be accepted from, will observe the changes you've made to yourself. They will observe your qualities, traits and character of the person they'd like to have. When they start to consider whether they should accept or deny you, your positive behavior will influence them to make a decision to favor you.

If, for instance, you're trying get someone to like you, don't appear as if you're trying to make yourself feel acceptable. Don't appear desperate or desperate. Instead, present yourself in a completely different way. You should appear as someone who is accepted. Your confidence will lead to the real happiness and success you deserve.

In anticipating the Yes that you anticipate, you build in yourself the image that is accepted in the mental image of someone who is disregarded. This is a crucial idea that you can apply even when you're not accepted. You'll realize that even if you're not accepted, you possess the capacity to be accepted, perhaps not today, but surely in the near future.

Fear of Rejection

The most damaging fears that could lead to rejection or hinder you from facing rejection head on fears is rejection in itself. It is crucial to remember that the fear of being rejected isn't something you should feel ashamed about. If you are afflicted by this fear be assured that you're not the only one with this anxiety. The fear of rejection isn't just widespread, but can also be traced back to the history of humanity.

The fear of being rejected is believed to stem from the human inclination that is rooted in the desire to feel a sense of belonging. When in the early days, people lived in members of a tribe or part of a group and felt a sense of belonging is extremely strong. This is due to the fact that in the time of tribalism, people could not afford to be excluded. people needed one another to survive, and one could not live on their own due to of the risks posed by wild animals or other tribes. If one is not part of his tribe expose themselves to dangers from people who don't belong or aren't recognized as part of the tribe.

This same urge persists even the present. Even in the present day the desire to be part of a group is just as powerful as it was a few thousand years ago. Instead of tribes, and methods for survival There are now groups that are both virtual and real as well as businesses, employment as well as other methods of living. Everyone regardless of age race, gender or other aspect of life, are afflicted by this fear. Only difference is how they deal with the fear of being rejected.

The two main ways people allow fear to influence them. The first is those who let fear impact them in a negative way. Certain people are so afraid about rejection, that their development is hindered. Always looking for safety they remain in their familiar areas. They only keep friends with those that are accepting of their company and are unwilling to look at different relationships that could allow them to grow yet still carry the possibility of rejection. Being a victim of worry will not lead you anywhere. It hinders you from becoming the person you're supposed to be. Additionally, the fear will never be gone, but it will linger within your mind until it is a part of your perspective in your daily life.

On the other side, there are people who make use of this anxiety to benefit others. If there's an anxiety, people utilize it to push them to better performance and relationships, as well as a more positive outlook on life. Instead of being a source of anxiety, fear becomes an anxiety-type thing which can lead to be more of a person. When you realize that there is a chance of rejection You will strive to be the best you can. To prevent rejection, or get rid of the fear of being rejected You devise strategies to ensure that it does not happen. The people who use anxiety not as a crutch but rather as a way to progress, are beneficial.

Be aware that the fear of rejection isn't an issue; it's normal and can be essential to allow you to grow. It's a plus when you can make use of it to realize your full potential , pushing you to the limit. On the other hand , in the event that you fail to utilize it in a appropriate way, it can be a hindrance that can hinder your progress.

Self-Approval

A single of the fundamental rules to adhere to when facing rejection is the notion of self-esteem. Although acceptance and belonging are vital in the world but it's by no is it the only thing that matters to be considered. Rejection is also a factor, but only to the extent that you don't resort to a constant desire for approval.

Also known as approval seeking behavior These are the behaviors you must be on the lookout for. The more you indulge in these behaviors, the more likely you will be on others to validate your self-worth and worth instead of you. There are many signs of the desire to always receive approbation from other people.

A few of them include:

Doing something that you're not expected or required to do simply because you don't want to say no yourself.

Let go of acts that have been committed against you in the belief that if they confront them, you'll lose their support

* Agreeing with concepts, discussions, or anything which you don't have a problem with in order to maintain the relationship

You are experiencing anxiety, stress, or anger whenever you dissatisfied with

* Always being gracious even when it is not necessary

* Proving that you are more knowledgeable than you actually do, but frightening that you'll be disapproved if the extent of your knowledge is revealed

* Disseminating falsehoods or facts that degrade or insult others in a way that they do not like others, and you are praised or are accepted

* Struggling to conform to or be accepted, by changing your character and values, beliefs, values or any other personal traits.

There are many other traits that could indicate an individual who aims to be liked at the at the expense of all other aspects about him. It is important to examine your own behavior or request an observation from others to determine if you exhibit these kinds of behaviors, and if they point towards an inclination to seek approval.

If you have these behaviors and you are prone to them, then do something to get rid of these behavior patterns by substituting them with self-acceptance or self-accreditation. There are many steps you can undertake to reach these goals in your the world:

Start by asking yourself simple , but extremely important questions. The answers to these questions can be found in the at-home privacy or deep within your thoughts. Try to answer them honestly as you can. Do you believe in your own self-worth? Do you require approval from others to feel confident about yourself? Do you self-judge yourself? And in the event that you do, how do you assess yourself?

If you discover that you have feel a lack of self-esteem, then you must change. Start letting away the idea that you require approval from others , and start by appreciating yourself first. Begin by feeling happy about yourself and celebrating your achievements and strengths. Remember the times you've stood your ground and been honest with yourself and accepted your own self. Remember how powerful those times were and draw inspiration from them as you seek self-acceptance.

Take the time to observe your own behavior for signs that suggest seeking approval. You can also ask the support of your circle of friends to assist you observe. Any time you observe yourself doing this change it immediately by using self-affirmation words.

Note that these periods of adjustment doesn't happen in a single day. If you've made an habit of these actions it may take a while before you are in a position to stop it. There is no excuse for putting off the task and the earlier you begin reviewing yourself and reversing these habits, the faster you can get rid of it.

Negotiation and Standing Your Stand

Negotiation is a strategy that you can employ when you're in the circumstance of being disqualified. If you feel there's still a chance to be accepted or that there is still time to argue your case to get approval Negotiation is among the most effective methods you can employ. It doesn't matter if you are couples trying to repair their relationship, are an employee who is trying to get the support of your boss, or selling a product and want to seal the deal, negotiation could make the different between rejection and acceptance.

There are many different negotiation methods readily available and are suitable for any situation of rejection. However, many of them follow the same fundamental principle. The negotiation steps you should master are:

* Recognizing your worth

* Slow and steady

* Plan the tactic

* Showing evidence

"Giving and taking"

Before entering into any negotiations to win acceptance, it is essential to be aware of the worth of the offer. If you're seeking acceptance for a product or service, it is essential to be aware of everything about what you're offering, not just its advantages or pros, but also its dangers and drawbacks. Make sure to negotiate slowly and nothing worthwhile can be achieved by rush. Take your the time to plan or prepare. In negotiations, be punctual to allow yourself time to think and pay attention to what the other side is talking about.

However it is crucial to design a strategy that fits the character of the other party. Don't use a standard approach to negotiations and identify the key areas of tension for the other party and what do they want to achieve as well as what characterizes him and what is the characteristics that he is most passionate about. If you know this information you can tailor your strategy to make the negotiation more successful. Bring along any evidence that can be able to support your arguments as a basis to reconsider or accept.

Remember that negotiation is not always about receiving something from a different party. Every relationship has a certain kind of exchange and negotiation. You must offer something in exchange to get the respect you desire. However put an amount you are able to and must offer.

Another strategy you could employ when you are rejected is to be firm. It is when you remain determined, confident, and don't take No as an answer. If you're convinced of your merit, the legitimacy of your concept and other aspects that need to be accepted and acceptance, then you are entitled to every right to continue.

Across Ages & Genders

It is possible that rejection is an universal issue, but every person reacts to it in a unique manner. There are certain patterns regarding the kind of response to rejection which can be attributed to an age-related aspect. Age groups of major importance, as shown in their maturity and emotional state can have a significant impact on the way people react to rejection.

These distinctions are important to be aware of because the more you understand how other people within your age range react, the more effectively you'll be able to deal with it. Apart from knowing your personal situation, you may also benefit from these suggestions about age-related differences with others.

One of the patterns that has been proven by research is that the more people age and gets older, the more anxiety about rejection is felt. It is because younger people can bounce back from rejection more easily in comparison to people of older age who are more difficult overcoming rejection. A study, for instance, was carried out that looked at the degree of pain felt by people aged between 18 and 26 and those who are 60 and over. Senior participants in the study were reported to be affected more severely when compared to junior participants.

Children

In the early years of childhood, the reasons for rejection are typically located in schools, as well as among groups of peers, neighbors sports teams and other similar groups. If you're an older sibling, parent or another adult who is accountable for the well-being of the child, you must be aware of the reasons behind rejection in the child's early years.

The first step to do is prepare yourself for the possibility of rejection from the child. Adults tend to respond to rejection from their children or others by referring to their own experiences of rejection in their past. In the process, they might unconsciously adopt the same coping strategies they utilized as were children. The danger with this approach is that it blocks the child from finding his own method of dealing with rejection. Furthermore, the setting in which you were rejected was very different today. As an example parents may struggle to give guidance to a child who is dissatisfied in the digital world for instance, through social media sites, even though she hasn't yet faced the same sort of rejection.

It is essential to ensure that when helping your child to overcome their fears, you do it with a clear, direct approach. Rejection from a club at school might not be a big deal to adults, but for a child, rejection could be among the most painful things the child imagines he will face throughout his life. If this happens, listen to your child and be sure that you take note of what he is saying is important to the perspective of his own subjective. Don't discount the experience and put in the same amount of effort as you would with any other kind of rejection.

If you can help your child cope with rejection, allow him to come up with his own methods, steps or strategies for overcoming rejection. Feeding your child spoons to help him overcome rejection will be less difficult, but only for a brief period. If you can you can help guide your child to equip himself with the tools needed to conquer rejection on his own. This will ensure that when we can grow up and having experiences from childhood which can aid him in coping.

Because of their lack of experience, kids are likely to have an idealized image of what is happening surrounding them. If they think that they're good at sports and think they are able to join the team. Be cautious when dealing with children. You need to control their expectations particularly when you notice that they're really keen about a sport. Bring them back to reality and encourage them to work harder to be part of the group or team.

Teenagers

The second important age group that is likely to bring the most turbulent years of the life of a person is who are teens. Changes in their bodies as well as in their minds, particularly the need to establish their identity and the most intense feeling of belonging. When a teenager discovers an organization to be part of it is likely that the teenage anxiety decreases. If however, any type of rejection occurs and it triggers intense anxiety.

If you're a teen or are looking to help adolescents overcome the fear of feelings of rejection, it is necessary to use an additional toolkit. For instance meditation, stress management , and expression of emotions can be beneficial for different kinds of age groups, however, for teenagers they can be ineffective, or even damaging. This is due to the fact that teenagers love the concept of autonomy. They want to accomplish things independently and without the help of adults. In the process of proving the ability to do things by themselves and without assistance, they may choose to reject assistance or even ignore the issue completely.

It is important to tailor your approach for teens who are disregarded. Some strategies you can employ include:

* Give them some space

* Be patient

Be aware of dangerous behaviour

Be open and willing for teenagers' conversations. Be sure to not glance over your shoulders all the time, instead let them have space. Rememberthat they enjoy being able to handle things on their own. Let them discover from mistakes and rejection. Teenagers have an ambiguity between helping them and intrusion. When they are readyto talk, teens will come up and seek your assistance. Be sure to remind them that you will be waiting and willing to listen whenever they're ready to discuss.

With outbursts and a sense of rebellion It is essential to have to have all of the patience have to help teens overcome their disapproval. There will be long moments of crying, loneliness and a refusal to communicate tempers, as well as various mood changes that challenge your patience. When this happens, you must keep yourself calm. If you must vent take it out of your home, so that your child isn't affected.

Although keeping your distance is beneficial but you must be aware of any dangerous behaviour. Teenagers who are known for their outbursts and unpredictable behaviour are more likely to channel their stress and other feelings into physically destructive behaviour. Watch out for those who stay out late into the evenings, and those who are becoming increasingly isolated or withdrawn from others.

One of the primary things you should examine is any physical changes that occur in their body. As an example, rejection could be extremely painful, and one solution to alleviate the stress caused by it is by the manifestation of it into physically damaging behaviors. The pain caused by the rejection can be temporarily replaced or covered up by the physical discomfort. Physical changes could refer to everything from weight issues self-inflicted wounds addiction to drugs and other destructive behaviours.

Be aware that these behavior should be addressed not just through themselves, but also by the root of their reason, which is rejection of the rejection itself. While you may treat the injury or change in diet but you must address the bigger issue in order to solve all issues once for all.

This doesn't suggest that adults who have matured and gained knowledge and wisdom gained from decades of experience, are in a position to overcome rejection with ease when compared to the younger generation. Although Part 1 and 2 of this guide is geared toward the needs of adults, there is a third step that could be required for those who are not.

Professional Support

Beyond the support from friends, family and loved ones, facing being rejected can become emotionally draining and psyche-related stress are the consequence. If this happens it is necessary to seek out professional help. Medical professionals, Life Coaches therapy professionals and others are needed to give adults, and other ages the scientifically-based care that is required.

Reactions to rejection can also vary according to the sex or gender individual. Research has shown that women experience more hormonal reactions when they are rejection is felt, which means women are more anxious by women in comparison to men. In spite of the findings, there is little research that shows a distinct different in the process of overcoming rejection between females and males. The majority of discussions are anecdotal in the nature of things.

Famous People who were rejected

Another method to overcome the fear of rejection is to learn from the many stories of success of people who have conquered the fear and challenges of rejection. They are renowned through their achievements and the acceptance of the communities they belong to as well as the world in which they reside. They are from every walk of life and backgrounds, as well as industries, and even the time.

Anna Wintour

Perhaps the most influential woman in fashion, Anna Wintour is the Editor-in-Chief for American Vogue. Under her direction the magazine has experienced unparalleled amounts of popularity. Her achievements are so impressive that she was appointed as the Creative Director for all of the publishing company. Her ideas and the company's are sought-after by famous fashion designers, celebrity magnates, politicians and other high-profile individuals.

In recognition of her numerous achievements and achievements, not only in fashion world, but also in the social and political circles She has been awarded numerous awards, like knighthoods of Great Britain.

It could be a bit surprising that she has derived her success not just from the accomplishments of others, but also from failings. Her most famous quote is saying, "I recommend that you all be fired. It's an excellent learning experience." Anna was fired in her role as the Junior Editor. If she had been able to ignore the rejection, she might not have achieved the level of success she is currently enjoying.

One thing that can take away from Anna is a unwavering belief in her abilities. Anna is aware of her worth as a person as well as professional. She carried confidence that those who were around her be drawn to and feel valued. If you're seeking approval from other people, try to be confident and believe in yourself.

Steve Jobs

Being fired from your job isn't a good thing, but being dismissed from your company could be even more damaging. In his final days, Steve Jobs is one of the most inventive and imaginative minds in the world today. Under his leadership, Apple, the company has revolutionized laptops, phones and computers , and is now introducing innovative technology. Apple is currently the most valuable companies worldwide, with revenues that are higher than that of whole nations.

While he is well-known as the chief executive of Apple however, there was a time in his professional career at which he was dismissed from his own company. Instead of lamenting about his despair or venting his anger, he channeled his determination to start an entirely new companycalled Pixar. This business went on to create some of the most well-known animated films, including Toy Story, Finding Nemo, Inside Out and the highly acclaimed Frozen and Minions.

When he returned back to Apple, Steve brought the company to new achievements and success. His design, his determination and passion for the company are evident in the products that are widely accepted around the world. One of the key lessons in overcoming the rejection of Steve was that he thrived off self acceptance, not on social acceptance. The media often quote him as declaring that Apple does not conduct market research. Instead, he is aware of what people want before they know they desire it. If Steve was completely dependent on what the customers would like from his designs, the Apple products might not be as popular like they are now.

Steven Spielberg

With 11 Emmy's, seven Globes as well as three Oscars, Steven Spielberg may be the most well-known director in Hollywood and maybe even the entire world. Under his supervision there have been a number of films which he has worked on in different roles are: Close Encounters of the Third Kind, Saving Private Ryan, Jaws, Jurassic Park, AI and the Indiana Jones series. His name is often associated with not only thought-provoking creativity in the genre of film, but also with the commercial success, profitability and global acceptance.

Before becoming the director he is now was, he attempted to attend the University of Southern California School of Theatre, Film and Television. He was rejected three times. Imagine someone as talented as

Steven being disqualified by the film school. Normal young adults seeking admission to colleges might be disappointed or even refusing to go back. Steven was not just trying to do it again, he repeated the process three times. This is another lesson to take away from this previously disregarded, but now successful people.

The ability to persevere and the determination are crucial for overcoming the fear of rejection. They are the traits you must have to keep your head upwards when you slip due to rejection. In like determination is crucial but you must also be aware of when it is time to make the decision to move on. Steven attempted to apply, but was denied and decided to apply to a different college. There he was accepted.

Sometimes, you have to stop for a moment, take a deep breath and think about all of possibilities. The ability to be persistent is admirable, but if is not used properly, it will keep you from success instead of bringing you close to it. Be flexible and change as necessary. Be open to all possibilities instead of being confined to one or two options. Your first choice might reject you , however the option which is the best choice for you might be able to accept you in the end.

Oprah Winfrey

The media mogul who is also a philanthropist awardee of the Presidential Medal of Freedom, holders of doctoral degrees and the most successful african-american billionaire U.S., Oprah Winfrey is another celebrity you can draw inspiration from. Her life is among the greatest examples of a the rags-to-riches story. She came from a poor family, and was the victim of several traumatizing events in her journey. From being sexually assaulted when she was nineteen, to the birth of an infant at the age of fourteen.

Despite the challenges She rose from journalist into a report, and eventually host of the show she created. In the end her media empire was growing and she gained acceptance across the globe by hosting her shows. Her views were valued her endorsements were received and her lifestyle was admired. But, despite her success, Oprah still had challenges.

The most talked about problems she had to face is her weight. People saw her weight fluctuated from being overweight, to becoming fit , only to gain the weight she had lost. Instead of turning to self-denial she adopted a totally different attitude. She confronted the problem head-on instead of hiding away from it.

This is a vital lesson to be learned in dealing with rejection. You must be aware of the value you have as a person and not make it a part of your weight. If a challenge are encountered, and when you're in danger of being judged by yourself or other people and you are unsure of your worth, it is important to admit it as something that is actually taking place. Nothing positive can be gained by denial of the truth. If you don't acknowledge it and the longer it takes you to heal from it, or, in this instance, overcome the rejection. There is no need to appear in public to show your concerns to the world. Instead, you can start by accepting the rejection yourself and working to resolve the problem and moving on.

Albert Einstein

The parents of his son say they were unable to talk to him until he was 4 years old. He also failed to read until seven. He was also expelled from school. One cannot imagine that the kid in this story was Albert Einstein himself. His name, frequently associated with innovation and creativity It is not often associated with failure or delay. But, these are the truths behind Albert's story.

Patience is a lesson that could be acquired from Albert. Acceptance is not always what you wish or when it is expected. Sometimes rejection may catch you off guard and make you feel awestruck. Acceptance might not happen in the span of a few months or a couple of years. Even in the event that you employ every trick to overcome rejection, this doesn't ensure acceptance.

The best thing one can accomplish is to just wait for acceptance to occur, however you must remain focused on the goal you want to achieve. The possibility of rejection will come at times, but it's usually only a few, or even several. But don't get scared or depressed by rejection. Instead, use it to improve your performance.

Refusing Others

A significant part of overcome rejection is to know how to despise other people. It is a lesson in empathy and giving back You also have to be able to effectively carry out the rejection in a way that people around you are able to have a positive perception of being rejected. One aspect that can greatly impact the process of beating rejection is the manner in which the rejection was handled.

Rejection is not always pleasant It can make people feel depressed, uneasy and even their hope. It can be a source of suffering both in the short as well as the long in the long run. However , all the anxiety and negative emotions can be diminished by delivering a rejection appropriately and with all the appropriate courtesies to soften the impact. If it's the person who you're disliking who will greatly benefit from how you handle the rejection, you also receive some benefits from it.

To eschew other methods, here are a few strategies:

Do not speak with an angry, emotional or agitated tone. Instead, be calm, calm and concise when you're refusing. People tend to imitate the way that they are treated by others and if you are taking an angry tone when you refuse the person, you'll most likely be treated the same.

Make use of a particular pattern of your body. Do not show signs of anxiety or discomfort for example, when you fidget, twitch or look in different directions. Instead, sit straight and straighten your back. Keep your arms by your sides, but not over your chest. Then, look straight in the eyes.

You can begin or put in a sentence, "I'm sorry" or "I apologize." It is in a manner of courtesy, therefore use them only sparingly. Avoid making too many excuses since if you do, someone will assume that you're feeling sorry and it is possible that your thoughts could change. Create sentences as concise as you can and do not use more words than you need to. The more concise the rejection the quicker you will escape from the situation.

It is perfectly acceptable to give an explanation as to as to why you're not able to accept the individual. Try to explain it as concisely as you are able to. Make sure you are honest and don't make up stories. Don't sugarcoat as it is only negative towards the other person. Do the best job you can, and do not give excuses for your actions.

One method to lessen the hurt further is to assist the person who was hurt by moving past the disappointment in itself. Instead of merely giving the rejection, offer alternative ways or opportunities for him to be appreciated. For instance, if you do not like the suggestion from your employees, provide constructive criticism instead telling them "No." The above actions will benefit you and the other party as you'll get better quality work in the next opportunity.

Be open to second opportunities. Don't be confined by being averse to people who you've rejected. This is not only harmful for the other person , but as well for you, since you might not be able to gain benefits once you've accepted another person.

When someone you've failed to accept attempts again to gain your acceptance, consider it with a fresh pair of eyes. You should definitely consider the first attempt at being accepted, but by evaluating the situation from a viewpoint. Don't use the initial rejection against another person instead, you can use it to evaluate the extent to which the other person has improved or changed and let that serve as your requirements for acceptance.

Chapter 9: A Clear Perspective

One of the best methods of making enemies is to directly critique or discredit the way that people perceive themselves. This makes sense since the majority people feel devalued when we feel that our self-image , which is to us similar to person we are a part of - is questioned. Most of us have been raised in a society of stories. Most people (and certain people greater than other) think of their lives as playing out as a novel or movie in which they are the main character. We create in our minds our own image that can be a star on the stage, regardless of how our physical appearance.

Ours is the lost princesses of an ancient and legendary kingdom. We are the orphan boy who is charged with the essential job of saving the planet. In other words in our personal opinion, we are remarkable individuals that do not merit this kind of conventional treatment, like being rejected from those who don't recognize us as the people we truly are.

Are you able to see the flaw with this photo? Everyone is too focused on being the most exceptional person ever to walk the earth. Nobody has the time to join in the hailing applause, cheering and cheers. In addition, nobody is waiting to see when you will finally achieve your goals. Some individuals might be looking forward to you falling onto your face, which would be one less pretentious for them. There are many intelligent people who say that the majority of the pain and sadness that we experience today stems from our desire to live our lives in a story-arc. This is why we all try to milk every moment in our regular life to the fullest extent it can bring. We need to practice to be ready for the moment when the "real" performance begins in the end, after all.

We all, regardless of whether we realize that or not are acting in a narrative and every one of us is a character. This is a fact that is easy to overlook, to our own disadvantage. If you step into the story of someone else and expect them to behave as side characters in the story of your life you will burn. To lessen not just the effect but also the incidences of being rejected in your own life, you must begin to accept the fact that the the world has a publication company. Everyone is eager to put their stories out there and you're bound to be sometimes trampled. Don't take the majority of it personally, it's not about your fault, and it's certainly not because you're not worthy of respect or love. The most disgusted individual on the planet is given a lot of love.

The fact that the person is entitled to the punishment or not is not the point. What matters is that regardless of how horrible he might appear to the majority of people, there are always people within the minority who know why he behaves what they see him. Do not be discouraged if the people around your now disapprove of you due to the fact that they don't "get" your perspective. The world is huge and there are 7 billion people living there; believe that at some point you will encounter people who understand your language and have the same lens. You could even become co-protagonists of comic book serial that is famous.

Rejection doesn't reflect your worthiness, however worthiness as well as"worthiness" as well as the "sales pitch" do not necessarily mean the same. All it comes down to is the way you view yourself, how you perform under that mindset and how people perceive your behavior on the way that their minds function. You might be a virtuous person within, but you could also be cautious: you aren't keen on letting your true self be seen because you believe that rub it into people's faces isn't good form However, a person who is watching you may take your polite and unassuming ways as being aloof - or even snobbery. And somewhere inside the brain's mechanism it could be transferred to untrustworthiness and immediately leading to the negative response towards you.

Some would argue that how people react to you is not your responsibility, being mindful about the gaps in your perception of yourself, to the way you conduct yourself and how someone else perceives your character to how they react - could affect your interactions with others. If the gaps can't be shut, then one should try to reduce these gaps.

Have ever wondered why individuals who excel in making friends aren't proficient at maintaining them? The problem isn't always their fault. However, two of the main reasons they usually contribute to are an over-complacency regarding the traits that draw people to them, and an inability to adjust to their changing relationships. It's true that the "there's no problem with me; you're the only one who's in trouble" mentality can derail an entire relationship before you could say. However, in these kinds of situations, rejection by force isn't the best course of decision anyone could consider. What both sides would like is for the other side to change even if they believe that they don't have anything about themselves that requires changing.

There is no way anyone is willing to hear they're in error on anything, particularly not when it means someone else is correct. The idea of being open to that possibility will require an amount of mental and emotional strength. It's an insane thought for many people, for instance: perhaps the reason why you keep being rejected is that the way you think is considered acceptable behavior in your own way can be offending to others. The most significant obstacle is your self-esteem. A few people would rather drown into a frozen lake rather instead of asking whether they were the one to blame for the incident or if they aren't willing to admit they've slipped up in some way.

A very significant lessons that a person can learn prior to advancing to maturity and deal with rejection more effectively is that he's not always correct. The opinions and perceptions of others would nearly always be in opposition to his however, that does not mean that they think differently but they think differently. In direct relation to that is it being possible that something you thinks of as rejection might not actually be a rejection in the slightest. What you may consider to be a deliberate decision to keep you out of something could actually be an error.

Your preferences make your inclusion in this particular group or event an issue, however the priorities of the other group could not be more different. And it is likely that you may want to be considered or even consider the decision to exclude yourself seriously never occurred to him. In contrast an "sudden" rejection could be communicated to you prior to the event as well, but because your preferences are very different from those of the other group All those warnings were ignored and not because you intentionally did not pay attention, but because you simply didn't think the need to.

If you find yourself replaying instances of rejection every time you encounter something similar to it, allow yourself to get sick of the routine. Most of the time it is just a matter of putting them away. keeps the memory fresh. Replaying a film that is bad over and over won't improve the quality of the film However, it will assist in dissociating you from the awfulness of the experience until it becomes just another movie.

In that moment you will be able to see the issue in a neutral way and maybe discover some hidden gems that the competing emotions have obscured. Every rejection of consequence is as if a message that is coded. The important information may not appear obvious initially, but when it is recognized as the most important source of information it is, breaking the code to discover the right message is the next step in one's journey to betterment. To do this all you require is a clear perspective.

Retrying and trying again

It's easy to imagine that being rejected in a work environment would not be as traumatic as personal rejection however, sometimes it can be more painful. The fact that you've had your skills discarded in favor of someone else's is personal when we insert our own ego into the process. It's hard to not suspect the possibility of foul play when, in our eyes, this appears to be the only plausible explanation. Be careful, it's okay to be angry, however, it's never acceptable to be unfair.

If your thoughts be dark every time you come across obstacles or obstacle, it could be that your ego has played a greater part in the events that led to the issue than you believed, and it could be the reason for your demise. Maintaining a positive attitude is crucial in a professional environment, especially when you're trying to make it into one. In an interview, candidates need to be mindful of their manner of conduct. Making it appear as if you're confident, self-assured and prepared to deal with unpredictable situations is great.

Confidence is not overflowing, and it's misplaced however it is not. Why? because interviewers have more in common with human beings than they appear to be. They can detect immaturity, emotions, or even nonsense from afar and are not able to handle it. Therefore, even though your professional credentials are in top in good shape, not many employers will not take the opportunity in the event that they believe they will never be in a position to count on your personal qualities.

However make sure to spend your time and effort on things that you are in control of. There's no way to make it easier when your applicants or colleagues have higher qualifications than you do at moment. It's not your fault that the interviewer you are interviewing with isn't at peace at the time you stumbled across the person, it's not a matter of luck if your novel you submitted was rejected due to the fact that they just purchased a book that's much or less like it.

The one thing you have to improve is your self. Polish or improve your skills and learn to understand people and situations more effectively Be more imaginative and avoid falling into the mistake of believing that the person you're currently is the most perfect version of yourself. And when you're doing that, you should return to the field and attempt again, this time from another angle. If you're willing to give it a few chances, eventually you'll discover the spot that can cause you to bounce up upwards, up, and up.

Neutralize Rejection

Then, there's love rejection. This is among the most difficult to deal with since love, which is the most powerful emotion in humankind is at play. For those who are who are rejected, it's of no use to claim that it was not their blame. The majority of people think that someone abandoned them or was unwilling to accept their feelings since there's something that's not right in them. What else could it be you think? Wrong. It's a tough lesson to master however it is a necessity to remember that no one should be a reason to make fun of. No one, and certainly never.

However it is equally crucial to recognize that there may be a legitimate reason (that is logic, however not necessarily "acceptable") that is behind the rejection that may remains hidden from you. It might or might not be directly connected to you or anything you've made or said, however the reason could be important to the person who is being rejected. It is important to respect their reasoning since if there's a that you do not want in addition to the pain that is bitterness. It's a highly useless exercise to figure out what the reason could be, and even more so to confront the individual with the issue.

Sometimes, they wouldn't have the ability to translate their feelings into words. The earlier you admit, with trust that there was no way you could have changed the situation in the past, the faster you could begin making decisions that take you forward. You've probably had a conversation with someone who could be referred to as masochistic if they keep repeating the same actions or reliving the experiences that brought him harm over the years. Don't be one of them.

If someone is your friend, you've likely faced the unenviable challenge of trying to advise him to take an approach that is different in the future. Your suggestions, naturally it was ignored. It's frustrating is and even although you may be able to understand the situation better today, it's still the fact that refusing to let go and refusing to give up are not productive actions. It is impossible for any person to aid someone who is committed to remaining in the position of a victim. In truth, very few would be willing to.

Before you start triggering a storm of disapproval from others you admire begin taking positive steps. Turn your emotional excess into physical exertion Keep your mind busy with stimulating material and most importantly of all, make your heartache of the past into a reservoir of helpful knowledge, not only for you, but to help others who may need it in the future. Being able to get advice in times in need is a nice thing as it makes you feel that others care about you. One way to top the positive feeling of receiving help could bring is to offer someone else assistance to them in return. There is no better method to beat the stigma of rejection than to help spread acceptance?

Chapter 10: Three Steps To Building Self-Confidence

Self-confidence is a crucial aspect for a person's daily life. Self-confidence means being confident and believing in your abilities. Learn to develop your self-confidence. Persistence is the key.

Many people experience self-confidence issues at one point or another. If this is the way you view yourself constantly, it could be detrimental. With a little help and direction you'll be on the path to breaking free of the trap of low self-confidence. It is possible to build confidence.

Step 1.) Develop A Positive Attitude

If you're looking to become positive about yourself and all the things you do, then you have to establish a positive mindset slowly, so that this attitude becomes automatic to you. Positive attitude doesn't suggest that you are apathetic. Your attitude will determine how you handle everyday challenges.

When you're in negative situations, the likelihood is that the surrounding will undermine your confidence and drag you down. Do not allow this to take place to your. It's your decision.

Because you are unable to alter the behaviour of other people or alter them, simply avoid them. Avoid separating yourself from people with negative attitudes. Make sure you are spending your time with the most positive people. Instead of spending half an hour with negative whiners and gossipers, you should spend just five minute with them. Don't be enticed by their negative thoughts listen to their thoughts. Look for those who are optimistic and spend an at least an hour or so with them for an hour. Their work will inspire you. Learn and take lessons from them.

Maintain a positive outlook towards a hostile work environment Do your best, avoid over-doing and blame others for not being able to assist you. Instead of trying to compete with others strive to think differently and become better than you were prior to. Always remember to take good care of yourself. Not eating lunch, taking breaks, working all day and the like is detrimental to you. It's about being positive towards yourself and the way that you live your life.

Accentuate your positive good qualities. Every morning, review all the things you've accomplished the previous day. Each night, you should sit down and record your accomplishments. It doesn't matter whether what you've accomplished is not significant.

We were all taught to dwell the negative aspects of life and it became a way of life. I am focused on the good and little events that happen to me. I am grateful for them and am proud of these events. Make sure you remember the positive things you've done. Learn more about stopping thinking about the negative.

Step 2.) Start A Physical Fitness Program

Integrate physical exercise in your daily routine. The physical exercise can provide you with feeling of achievement and a sense of self-worth. It helps get rid of any negative thoughts.

For me , exercise is one of the best methods to overcome self-doubt. After exercising, I feel great and more confident. Most important, my posture improves. If you exercise, your body produces endorphins which help to reduce anxiety and can alter your mood.3 Exercise gives you a feeling of satisfaction and enhances your self-esteem. You'll feel confident about yourself, and it makes you feel happy.

Step 3: Create goals that are achievable

Set yourself some goals. Write down what you'd like to achieve and then work towards each target one at a time and when you reach them, feel proud of your achievement. A goal is a way to define a particular goal and makes it in the forefront of your head. Set goals and reach them will show you (and in turn, in your mind's subconscious) that you've succeeded and, as a result you will gain confidence in yourself.

Nothing is more important when it comes to goal setting than having a clear idea about what you want to accomplish or attain. If you are uncertain about this, or you're unsure it is unlikely that you can achieve what you want.

How to set your objectives

1. Once you have a clear idea of your goals, you can note it down with a positive and specific tone. Instead of writing "I will exercise more often," compose "I will exercise four times a every week.". Do you see that the second choice is clearer and more precise than the first? It provides you with a concrete goal to be able to achieve, not an abstract idea to think about.

2. After you've determined the goals you want to achieve adhere to the goals. Consider it to be one of the most important aspects of your life to achieve the goals you have set.

3. Be sure to keep track of your goals and note the achievements you've made to assess how far you've made it When you've reached your goals then you should reward yourself.

Setting goals and demanding of yourself that you achieve or exceed your goals is essential to success in your life. The goals you set may be either long or short-term.

Certain goals are either frequently or weekly, whereas some are annually scheduled and some are in the future. They are the ones you are aiming for, as archers aiming at the bull's eye of his target. Remember: If you are aiming at nothing, this is exactly the target you'll hit.

Get rid of past memories. The past is over. There's nothing you can do to remedy negative past experiences. If you did make mistakes or think that you did something wrong, learn from the experience, work on improving and proceed.

Use any of the suggestions to your daily routine. This will allow you build confidence in yourself. The more you conquer life's obstacles, the more you can believe in yourself, and you will change your perspective.

Don't hold off until everything is perfect. It's never going to be perfect. It will be obstacles as well as obstacles, and even less than perfect conditions.

How to Improve Your Self-Confidence

Confidence is defined as the perception of one's capabilities based depending on the situations. A belief or faith that one will act in a proper and efficient manner. The ability to be certain. The process of building confidence involves shifting perceptions and expectations.

The confidence we have in ourselves is based on how we have performed in similar situations. We judge the situation based on reflections and comparisons. These comparisons result from conclusions regarding past accomplishments family members, parents, friends and other authority figures. The way you have performed in the past makes us feel confident.

The four steps you must take to increase your self-confidence are:

1. Stop striving for perfection and accept that the information you received was not always the truth. Be focused to your best

qualities and greatest abilities and perform your best. Begin to learn ways to communicate yourself more confidently methods to increase your confidence.

2. Spend time with positive people. Consider the those you spend time with. If they're always slamming you spend more time with those who aren't.

3. Each time you feel like you have failed, make it an opportunity to learn. Don't be worried that you'll be a failure. Failure isn't a thing; rather you're trying towards doing things differently.

4. Be kind to yourself. Do the best you can for yourself and give yourself respect and love.

You can't change the world around for you, but you are able to take charge of the way you feel. Be aware of your inner dialogue and practice assertiveness. Make use of introspection, and more time in silence, allowing yourself to see the wounds from your past that aren't healed yet.

Tip #1 1. Rely on your own self-evaluation

Do not give your power away to other people. Be aware of what you feel. Build a relationship of love with yourself. Believe in your own intuition, and in your strengths. It is not possible to be self-confident every day But you are able to change and grow. Do not worry about the opinions of other people. This was the most difficult lesson I've had to take on. I was always looking for approval. I have now realized that the other's opinions are just that.

Stop worrying all day about how others feel. Everyone has their own opinions and different capabilities. Therefore, you need to concentrate on your strengths and strengths. Be your own personal most trusted friend. Give yourself a hug and patience. The way you conduct yourself will be more significant than skills and can help you feel more confident.

Tip # 2: Change your negative inner-dialog

Sometimes, this negativity could hinder you from trying something you really want to do. When you are aware of this negative idea, alter the thought. Remind yourself that you are grateful. In this way, your negative inner dialogue will try to shield your. Be sure to always replace your negative thoughts by a positive affirmation.

Enhance your inner-talk and increase your self-confidence. My inner dialogue was full of criticism since I was raised by perfect parents. It took me a long time to be able to accept myself, until I was able to overcome the majority of my negative thoughts so that I could feel like an enthused person.

Have you ever had the experience of making a mistake, and then thinking: "I am a stupid. I'll never be able to do this correctly, so there's no reason to persisting.". Pay attention to what you're telling yourself. Then, you can choose to end it or continue forward or talk to that portion of yourself which is causing you to feel defeated and affirm: "Thank you for sharing I am aware that I did make a mistake, but this is a great way to improve. When I am aware of the mistake I made, I'm able to try again. A mistake made by me doesn't mean I'm a fool."

A positive inner-dialogue can help to boost confidence in yourself. Your confidence is affected by how you talk to yourself. Make a conscious effort to speak to yourself more positively.

Tip #3: Alternate your posture

It is crucial to be aware of how your body's physiology affects your confidence levels. You can make use of your physiology in order to build confidence. Change your posture to lifting your head and your shoulders back. smile, and keep eye contact.

Anthony Robins says that emotion is generated by motion. Everything we experience comes from how we utilize our bodies. Therefore, if you consistently lift your shoulders, and walk as if you're exhausted and tired, you'll feel tired.

Do some standing exercises and walk with your head raised. Look people in the eye. Your body language will determine what people will be able to tell. A good posture can make your feel more secure, and people will see that you are confident and self-assured.

Positive affirmations to build self confidence

Re-programme your mind's subconscious to be more confident and eliminate negative habits and thoughts. Affirmations are positive words that are used to define a desired event the course of action or the situation. They are often repeated to impress your mind.

1.

Do these affirmations for at minimum 21 days. You may choose to practice at least one day per every day for a minimum of. Don't miss a day. should you fail, you can start the process over. The affirmations can be said in front of others or record them in a notebook. If you are able to say the affirmations out loud, repeat them in the mirror in front of you and repeat them 10 times. If you decide to record them make each one of them a note 10 times.

* I am confident in myself

"I am very proud of me

* I'm able to accomplish anything I want to accomplish

* I am competent and strong

* I am an award-winning winner

Everyday in all ways, I feel ever more confident.

* I have faith in all situations

* I believe in myself

* I believe of my capabilities

* I am confident in myself

* I have earned the right to be successful

* I acknowledge who I am.

My future is decided by me

* I am competent and smart

My body language reflects confidence

* I radiate confidence.

* I transform negative situations into positive ones

" I'm a person who is positive

My confidence is constantly increasing

* I am confident and certain

Fear of affirmations that criticize

*I accept me as what I am, and am not afraid to face criticism from other people

* I value myself.

Affirmations about inferiority

* I am satisfied with myself and feel very happy about myself

"I'm a adored and loved and

A lack of assertiveness is a positive affirmation.

My assertiveness improves my relationships

* I am comfortable with my choices

The perfectionism affirmations

It's okay to make mistakes

* I don't need the perfect score. My best is sufficient.

Affirmations of insecurity

*I trust in my intuition over all else.

* I am that I am not having any knowledge.

Fear of affirmations about rejection

* I am no longer frightened of my fear of being rejected

Conclusion

Rejection is never an enjoyable experience for anyone. It is denying your desire of being loved by and appreciated by people. However, rejection is a sad aspect of life. It is not a good idea to let it define youor not risk anything and never move your life even further. You'll keep yourself in the confines of your anxiety.

Once the initial pain of rejection wears off and you are able to back to your feet. Don't allow the fear of hurt keep you inside a shell. It is time to break free from your shell and go the world by storm, either regardless of rejection.

Life isn't designed to be lived with security. It is possible to create your own bubble, in which you do not consider the possibility of being disqualified. However, you are missing numerous opportunities in which you could be welcomed. Your ideas and hopes aren't going to get a chance to shine If you are shut away from the world due to anxiety.

The hurt of rejection isn't worth the suffering of a lifetime of regrets. Consider taking some of the biggest chances that can make your life go around. You'll never know whether something will turn more efficiently than you have imagined until you attempt.

With this book as a guide and a starting point, you can work to conquer fears of rejection. Don't be afraid and begin living your life. If you've got an idea, novel or screenplay, or someone you'd like to approach take it to the next level. You might get a no. If you receive an answer, it's simply a chance to improve and go on to the next thing that is great that you will experience. A person's decision to reject you doesn't reflect on your character. Some other person could welcome your thoughts or ideas with welcoming arms.

The fear of rejection shouldn't hinder you from pursuing your dreams. You must embrace the world. Be adventurous. Take a chance to try new things. Create yourself a rejection-proof person so that rejection doesn't bounce off you and doesn't stop you from living fully. The concepts in this book will assist you in becoming unstoppable and where rejection will not hold you back.

www.ingramcontent.com/pod-product-compliance
Lightning Source LLC
Chambersburg PA
CBHW060330030426
42336CB00011B/1284